GUT FEELINGS:

SOCIAL AND EMOTIONAL STRUGGLES WITH CROHN'S AND ULCERATIVE COLITIS

BY LINDA KRIGER

FINDING FREEDOM FROM SHAME AND ISOLATION

First published by Dog Ear Publishing
4011 Vincennes Rd
Indianapolis, IN 46268
www.dogearpublishing.net

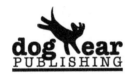

ISBN: 978-1-4575-3940-4

This book is printed on acid-free paper.

Printed in the United States of America

To my husband, Jake, whose love has been strong and unchanging and whose patience and support made it possible to bring this book to life.

"From this small beginning, we have witnessed the evolution of a Frankenstein monster that, if not threatening to life, frequently results in serious illness, often prolonged and debilitating."

— Dr. Burrill Crohn and Dr Harry Yarnis, *Regional Ileitis*, 1957

Table of Contents

Introduction

While waiting in line for a glass of wine at a large fundraising event, I fell into conversation with a woman who asked what I did for a living. When I told her I was a writer, she asked what I was writing. I said I was researching a book about the social and emotional impact of inflammatory bowel disease (IBD) on people under 30. She asked why I had chosen that topic. Years earlier, I would have deflected the question with a nondescript reason to avoid answering truthfully, but I had come to grips with the fact that secrets are toxic, so, internally, I took a deep breath and replied that I had had ulcerative colitis and my entire colon had been removed and replaced with a J-pouch to substitute for my large intestine.

The next thing I knew, she disappeared. I stood there, contemplating the awkwardness of the moment. Our brief conversation highlighted one of the central issues I address in *Gut Feelings*: Speak about my condition and I may alienate my listener. Don't speak about it and I stifle who I am and what I have gone through.

Issues related to inflammatory bowel disease are very real for the 5 million people worldwide and 1.6 million people in the United States with Crohn's disease and ulcerative colitis, which comprise IBD. If you have IBD, you may live with blood and pus in the toilet, frequent cramps, stomach and joint pain, skin eruptions, bloating, weight loss, and lethargy. You must decide how to navigate the world of seemingly healthy people. You must also formulate in each moment how much to tell people about the cause of your symptoms to minimize the risk of turning someone off, as I obviously did in that brief interaction.

Being frank about their medical condition is not an issue for young people with cancer, asthma, diabetes, or, for that matter, any other chronic disease. But talk openly, even with friends, about why you scope out bathrooms everywhere, why you avoid going outside your home for fear of having an accident in your pants, or what the real reason is behind your quitting the school soccer team, and you run the risk that the conversation will dissolve abruptly into awkward, helpless silence or, worse, pity.

Cultural Attitudes Toward Feces

Write what you know. That is the standard advice to writers. I know about being a teenager and someone in her 20s and 30s with runaway ulcerative colitis. Although I didn't become symptomatic until I was almost 16, I also know about living in an antagonistic relationship with defecation from my earliest years. I remained silent about it because I was a child and I didn't know how to articulate what was going on with my gut. And also, what friend wants to hear about my severe constipation?

Secrecy and shame around defecation are such cultural norms, so ingrained in all of us, that we don't question them or even think about them. After all, what separates humans in Western culture from other animals, in part, is that we defecate behind a closed door. What goes on in the bathroom is private and distasteful and it is never mentioned in conversation except as a spontaneous expletive.

But, as it turns out, it wasn't always that way. In their book *End Product: The First Taboo*, Dan Sabbath and Mandel

Hall write that we are not born with repulsion toward feces. They cite three physicians from the University of Pennsylvania who studied reactions to body odors. They discovered that four-fifths of the 3-year-olds in their study found the smell of feces pleasant. Only an eighth of the adults liked the odor. This is not to say that we should feel guilty for finding fecal odors repugnant. But the feelings we take for granted did not always exist. We can only acknowledge the conceivable damage they can do to people whose disease centers around feces.

The presence of shame and disgust about defecation in general and IBD in particular reminds me of the time, not so long ago, when women with breast cancer couldn't utter the word "breast" in public because it was so shocking. Newspapers were complicit. When breast cancer patients died, as they often did in those days, obituaries simply said they died from cancer. Fortunately, the taboo over the word "breast" has dissipated, and my hope is that, one day, the same will be true of the words surrounding defecation.

The taboo around excretion will be difficult to overcome, but to date, so many taboos have been freed from the constraints of silence, there is no reason to believe it won't happen regarding the body's elimination system, too. However long that takes, the embarrassment associated with IBD must be confronted now. That is a central aim of *Gut Feelings*, to tackle the destructive impact that taboos regarding IBD impose on those of us with the disease, particularly with regard to our social, psychological and emotional lives.

How This Book Can Help You

For years, the best advice that IBD advocates have offered in books and on the Internet are cheerleading messages that say, in effect, "Yes, it's hard to have IBD, but you can do it." Having lived through the physical and psychic pain of ulcerative colitis, I have found scant comfort in these words. The messages seemed simplistic. They skimmed the surface of a complex cauldron of emotions that young people experience with IBD. In retrospect, I have to acknowledge that in the course of researching this book, I've come to understand that the positive, cheerful message I used to disparage is actually true. Living with IBD is hard, and it is also true that you will get through it. But that is only the beginning of the discussion.

I felt the book had yet to be written that seriously examined the emotional roller coaster experienced by people with IBD. I was curious to hear patients describe how they responded to their disease and how IBD had transformed their lives for better or for worse. The stories I heard moved me. I listened to many iterations of how parents and young people were dealing with the long haul, how they were gathering their emotional and psychological resources and struggling with their new normal.

My hope is that patients, parents, siblings, and significant others will feel solidarity with people in the book. If a book like *Gut Feelings* had existed when I was diagnosed with ulcerative colitis, I would like to think my early life would have been much easier. I would have felt camaraderie with other young IBD patients. At least I would have known they existed, which I did not. My parents might have found common ground with other parents, observed how they responded to their children and, perhaps, they would have been less critical of me for having developed the disease.

Many books about IBD are focused on physical symptoms, including those that offer prescriptive advice on ways to alleviate your distress with special diets, yoga, and herbs. This is not one of those books. While I will take you through patients' difficulties in getting diagnosed, dealing with medications and exploring nonmedical approaches, I will examine these largely through a psychological, social, and emotional lens, so that you can use the book as a compass for your own experience. My hope is that you will learn how people under age 30 have coped with all the complicated aspects of growing up while juggling the complexities of IBD.

Gut Feelings delves into the interior lives of people with IBD. Issues include dealing with schoolmates, teachers, and administrators; talking about your disease and getting support; handling food and alcohol in social situations; navigating the dynamics with parents and siblings; and handling depression, stress, dating, and work life.

Patients Expose Their Interior Lives

To understand the diverse ways in which people under age 30 are grappling with IBD, I interviewed more than 100 young people, along with many of their parents, siblings, and romantic partners. I found them on Facebook, in Internet chat rooms, and through word of mouth. After telling me how they had been diagnosed — often a long, complicated account — they spoke in detail about the emotional and social effects of IBD on their lives. At the end of each interview, I also asked them to identify the upsides of IBD, that is, how their lives have been transformed for the better because of it. After sometimes pausing several moments to think about this new way to look at their disease, almost everyone was able to find positive contributions that having IBD had made to their lives.

Understandably, some people preferred to protect their privacy when they spoke frankly about intimate issues and relationships, so I decided to use first names or pseudonyms for everyone. I am deeply grateful to people who discussed tender and raw emotions as they spoke about the complications that IBD had inflicted on their lives.

CONCLUSION

To date, no key has been found that will unlock the puzzle for everyone with IBD. Just as there is no one cure for cancer, it appears that each patient's IBD throws out symptoms with various degrees of severity and different responsiveness to treatments. For example, I have had virtually no problems with my J-pouch, whereas other patients must be hospitalized multiple times to cope with chronic inflammation and other complications.

Immunological diseases like IBD pose monumental challenges for researchers and clinicians. As one patient pointed out, people with IBD all come from different families, with different genetic legacies and different psychological circumstances. It is up to each of us to find the path through the thicket of illness and move toward open ground, where we can find some semblance of peace.

It is my keen desire that *Gut Feelings* will assist patients and those who love them in identifying with and learning about how others deal with their disease. I am thankful to the many people who opened their hearts and spilled their guts to me. I was gratified when several patients expressed appreciation for the opportunity to tell their story. They said it was the first time they had traced the arc of their entire experience, not just medically, but emotionally and psychologically. It was healing for them to do so. They spoke in the hope that sharing their experiences would ease the stress on others in coping emotionally and physically with IBD. Each patient's experience was distinctive, indicating to me that each case of IBD is somewhat different from everyone else's. I did find one common denominator among all the patients I interviewed: Everyone was searching for understanding and compassion.

CHAPTER ONE
Being Young With IBD

As sympathetic about your suffering as people may be, anyone who has not had to cope with IBD cannot understand all the layers of turmoil that those with IBD have gone through. So, at the outset of this book, I offer you the story of my own emotional and psychological experience with ulcerative colitis, not because my case is unusual or important (except to me), but because my story contains many elements with which you may resonate. In fact, many of you have experienced far worse physical symptoms. I was never hospitalized with colitis, and I lost only two weeks of work because of it. However, the psychological toll and emotional agitation it caused me are shared by many of you, no matter the level of your physical illness.

My Story

I don't remember a time when I had a friendly relationship with the toilet. From early childhood, my mother firmly insisted that I sit until I moved my bowels. For long stretches of days, nothing budged. I endured frequent suppositories and old-fashioned enemas. I still see the red rubber bag hanging from the bathtub curtain rod with a tube running down, inserted into my bottom while I bent over the tub. Even as a young child, although I couldn't put words to it, I felt humiliated, utterly stripped of power over my body, very much the same way I felt years later from ulcerative colitis.

When I was 15, blood began appearing in the toilet bowl. First, it showed up on the hard stool as a few warning specks that I discounted as caused by straining and irritation. Then, one day, the blood ominously colored the bowl red. For weeks, I didn't tell my mother, out of shame and an attempt to maintain my privacy. Finally, when the bleeding continued and intensified, mixing with pus, I broke down and spoke up. The doctor called it proctitis, an inflammation near the rectum, and he put me on the medication I would take for more than 30 years. Sometime later, my diagnosis was upgraded to colitis on my descending colon. By the time my colon was removed, ulcers had engulfed the entire organ.

During the next several years, I had plenty of stress during my academic life. While colitis was a reality in my life during college and journalism school, it didn't take center stage, which calls into question the degree to which stress and symptoms always go together. My symptoms were kept in check by medication. I mostly struggled with continuous constipation.

My relationship with my mother, always difficult, was further complicated by my colitis. At the time, ulcerative colitis was not yet understood to be an autoimmune disorder, so, without any information to prove otherwise, my mother asserted that I could banish the disease if only I would eat better. My father joined her in this, and he was furious that I ate sushi, a new exotic food in America then, certain that the raw fish was terrible for my gut. It's true that I ate what I liked. At work, we grabbed cheeseburgers and fries for lunch. I didn't have the will power to eat differently.

In my late 20s, I began to develop more serious symptoms. Bleeding from my rectum intensified and my red-blood-cell count plummeted. I had severe stomach cramps and an almost constant, strong urge to evacuate. I took a leave of absence from my job and returned to my parents' home in Connecticut to rest. I felt depressed, utterly desolate, without support, and alone.

In fact, I *was* isolated. I had never known anyone else with colitis. These were the days before the Internet and the Crohn's and Colitis Foundation of America (CCFA) had extended its reach into communities around the country. Now there are IBD chat rooms, IBD support groups, IBD blogs, IBD summer camps, and CCFA-sponsored education days at hospitals, all of which would have helped my family to better understand the disease.

I returned to work feeling rested, but still physically compromised. Ulcerative colitis dominated my life, creating complicated feelings about my body. I dated a little, but I was terrified of having an accident and having to run to the bathroom. Colitis was beginning to be my constant companion, leaving little room for anything else but my job. I lost 20 pounds in a month.

My life was transformed after a colleague, who undoubtedly suspected I had developed anorexia, did me a great favor and referred me to her therapist. In a space where it was safe to unleash all the anger and grief I'd held inside since childhood, I began, over the next six years, to feel more psychologically whole. At the same time, my physical condition began to stabilize.

In the midst of this inner physical and emotional turmoil, I decided to take over the medical beat at the paper I wrote for. I had experienced how little the pharmaceutical and medical professions had to offer to alleviate my symptoms, much less cure my disease. And I had come to see how chronic diseases challenge Western medicine. For six years, until I quit daily journalism, I worked energetically as a medical writer, writing, in part, about the dilemmas doctors coped with when faced with intractable chronic illness.

Events in my life spiraled forward quickly, creating upheaval, whether they were personally shattering or joyful. Without communicating their plans to me, my parents moved to within ten minutes of my home. Then, my father died. Over the next years, I met my first husband; we married; my mother died; I gave birth to two sons; and I divorced my husband, leaving me a single mother of an 8-month-old and a 3-year-old. Through it all, my colitis stayed fairly consistent, even getting a little better — another instance in which my stress levels didn't correlate with my symptoms.

Although my colitis was stabilized, I didn't take my relative good health for granted. I continued to take the maximum dose of Azulfadine, a sulfa drug used to treat ulcerative colitis, every day. Every night, I forced down psyllium seed, which was then a grainy, gelatinous stool softener mixed with water, which kept my colitis at the front of my consciousness, even as it receded to the background of daily life. (I hear they've since improved the consistency.) Soon, I met a wonderful man whom I loved and who loved me. I was finally and completely happy.

Still, because I had spent decades living with an inflamed colon, the chances that rogue cells would pop up put me at a heightened risk for colon cancer. Although I'd had many benign polyps removed over the years, a greater danger was posed by abnormal and potentially precancerous tissue (called dysplasia) that lies flat against the wall of the intestine. Suddenly, after many successful colonoscopies, the results weren't so good. In the late '90s, my doctors discovered dysplasia in my colon, although they failed to explain to me the implications of its re-growth in a single spot. One spring day in 2000, after my most recent colonoscopy, I got a call telling me that my entire colon had to be removed to prevent imminent colon cancer.

I felt defeated. At 49, I had the hubris to imagine I'd beaten colitis. I hadn't bled rectally for nearly a decade, nor had I felt any urgency to run to the bathroom. Still, the reality of my present situation was undeniable. Without the surgery, I almost certainly faced colon cancer. With the surgery, I faced an uncertain future with a J-pouch. But at least I would have a future and my little boys would have their mother. In fact, I put their adorable, wallet-sized photographs on the surgeon's desk at our interview and told him that if I died on the operating table, "You get them."

Afterward, in the small, curtained-off recovery area where I was parked after the surgery, through the blur of anesthesia I heard that my entire colon had looked like a battlefield. Of course, I thought. I *knew* that a civil war had been waging inside my body for years.

Three months later came the second surgery. A J-pouch, an internal kind of mini-colon reservoir fashioned from the last 12 inches of my small intestine, was attached to my anal muscles so I could go to the bathroom like everyone else. Two weeks after surgery, I was in my backyard barbecuing hamburgers. True, I had to go back to the hospital with a bowel obstruction because I was doing too much too soon, but I was ready to move on with my life.

Many people with a J-pouch suffer from an inflamed pouch, called pouchitis, which causes many of the same symptoms as colitis. However, I've been virtually problem free for more than a decade post-surgery. After all those years of putting up with rock-solid stools, I revel that they are now liquid and just slide out of me. I have gone through good times and not-so-good times with my J-pouch, but I am thankful that I have never needed to be hospitalized or treated for pouchitis. I know that others are not so lucky.

Since the surgery, I eat and drink everything and take no medication. And yet, despite my good fortune, I can't shake the habit of worrying about ill health: How long will my J-pouch remain functional? Will I suffer intestinal obstructions as I age? Will I develop anal cancer one day? Will my luck run out and afflict me with severe bouts of pouchitis? The specter of ulcerative colitis hangs over me. I am rid of the disease. I may never rid myself of the lingering dread.

Being Young with IBD

Having been a young person with IBD, I am particularly sensitive to the way the disease compounds insecurities and self-consciousness. Growing up is difficult enough under the best of circumstances. Being a child, an adolescent, or a young adult isn't just about joyous abandon, although there is plenty of that. Being young also involves struggles with anxiety, inhibition, and inner turmoil. Your identity is being shaped. Even without the added complications of illness, friendships and cliques come and go. Grades go up and down. Girls reject and boys leave. Jobs are won and lost.

Youth is a time to stick your toe into the water, even when you don't know what will happen when you do. I love the biblical allegory about the parting of the Red Sea during the Exodus, which reminds me of this uncertain time of our lives. According to legend, a man named Nachshon was the first Israelite to enter the sea, while the others cowered on the shore. He walked farther and farther into the sea until the water reached his nose. Only then did the Red Sea part. It sometimes feels that way when you're young (sometimes when you're not so young, too.) Many social situations feel risky and dangerous. When you are feeling emotionally vulnerable, whether you are a child, a young person, or an adult, the challenge is to wake up every morning and summon the courage to walk out the door and plunge into life. How much greater is the challenge if you have Crohn's disease or ulcerative colitis.

The first thing to know about having IBD when you are young is that you are far from alone. Tens of thousands are diagnosed with Crohn's disease or ulcerative colitis between the ages of 15 and 35; some are children as young as 2 years old. The most common age of onset for Crohn's is between 15 and 30. The most common age for the onset of ulcerative colitis is between 15 and 25. (Centers for Disease Control and Prevention, 2014)

Children under 18 are the fastest-growing patient population, according to the CCFA. Inflammatory bowel disease (IBD) affects 71 in 100,000 children in the United States (43 per 100,000 children with Crohn's disease and 28 per 100,000 children with ulcerative colitis), and approximately 25 percent of all individuals with IBD are diagnosed during childhood or adolescence. Several studies indicate that cases of IBD are rapidly increasing among children and teenagers, according to Dr. Lee "Ted" Densen, medical director of Cincinnati's Children's Hospital Medical Center's Inflammatory Bowel Disease Center. No one knows the reason. One in five children diagnosed with IBD present with severe disease. In milder cases, symptoms can include stomach pain, diarrhea, and constipation. In more severe cases, they can consist of fatigue, diarrhea, bleeding, fistulas, infections, and ancillary conditions, including joint pain and rheumatoid arthritis, another autoimmune disorder.

Why Focus on Young People?

As I suggested in the introduction, there has been little in-depth exploration of the psychosocial experiences of young people with IBD, or, for that matter, adults with IBD. Still, I chose to focus on young people because my memories of my own youth remain poignant and rich, as painful as they were. IBD pushed me out of the emotional rut I'd fallen into. I had displayed the emblematic features of someone with IBD: I internalized stress and put on a good face. I began to appreciate the fact that despite all the genetic and, perhaps, environmental factors that had led me to develop colitis — all those cheeseburgers and fries for example — there were emotional and psychological features as well. My colon was my body's vulnerable place, wherein resided all the tension, grief, and disappointment of my early years. Perhaps I could have developed migraines, but that wasn't where I was susceptible.

I decided to write this book because I knew others with IBD had their own stories to tell about how they and their families were handling the disease and what they'd learned about life with Crohn's disease and ulcerative colitis. The interviews affirm that IBD interferes with all the fragile undertakings of youth. It barges into daily life like a nasty, uninvited guest. It can limit activities, complicate friendships and romantic relationships, and create dependency on parents at a time when individuation — the act of becoming an independent individual — normally occurs. Every aspect of existence becomes subtly or overtly skewed in school, in the workplace, in traveling, and in dating.

To get a sense of what it's like to be young with IBD, imagine a group of 9-year-old girls in the fourth grade who scrawl the words "fat" and "cow" on a classmate's desk when she comes to school with distended cheeks. She has to take the steroid Prednisone to control rampant ulcerative colitis, despite the side effects. A ninth grader with Crohn's disease is bullied after his stepbrother tells friends that the boy had a colonoscopy, which involved having a scope pushed up his rear end. A 28-year-old man who already had problems with dating is enveloped in self-doubt after colon surgery leaves him with a colostomy bag.

Another aspect of living with IBD in your youth is that intimations of mortality may intrude, which we usually associate only with childhood cancers. Gina, who was 26 when we spoke about her life with Crohn's disease, talked about her mortality in a way few people her age normally would. "We all think about death and dying all the time, not because we want to or because we're suicidal," she said in the matter-of-fact tone of someone who has spent years acquiring self-acceptance. "We think about death because we have a chronic illness. Yes, I have a living will. We have our bucket list. That's realistic."

Parents of children and teenagers with IBD feel helpless, frustrated, guilty, and worried. Some become familial cops, checking whether their children have taken their medications and whether they should be eating that piece of pizza, worried that their children are poor guardians of their own health.

Other parents know deep down that the best they can offer is love, advocacy, and support through the devastating low times, watching their beloved children flounder, hoping that they will find their way to self-care, and knowing that sometimes the best care isn't enough against an insidious, persistent disease. The spouses, boyfriends, and girlfriends of older patients often learn to accept the limitations that the disease imposes on their loved ones and on their lives together.

Among those who suffer with IBD, I'm one of the lucky ones, as my story indicates. But although my suffering was relatively lighter than that of some, I know intimately the universal heartaches and headaches of young people caused by the emotional and physical pain of IBD. Parents, physicians, and young people can benefit from a vivid understanding of how IBD intensifies the normal emotional hardships of youth almost to the breaking point. The deeper your insight, the better you will be able to cope with IBD's challenges and move along with endurance and fortitude.

CHAPTER TWO
IBD: Fact And Speculation

If you are under 30 and have inflammatory bowel disease (IBD), you know what it is and how it feels. But if you are new to IBD or are reading this book to learn more about the inner life of someone you know with IBD, here is a brief primer on the disease. We begin with a common misperception.

IBD, which comprises Crohn's disease and ulcerative colitis, is often confused with irritable bowel syndrome (IBS), a troublesome but less biologically invasive condition. Many people with IBS assume that they know what it's like to have stomach problems and they often believe that their suffering is similar to that of those with IBD. So it is important to make a clear distinction between the two.

Irritable bowel syndrome, also known as spastic colon, is ubiquitous. One in six Americans complains of abdominal pain, cramping, gas, diarrhea, and constipation. But as annoying and disruptive as IBS is, the structure of the intestines remains normal. It is thought that signals go back and forth between the stressed brain and the bowels and cause extremely uncomfortable symptoms. IBS can be controlled by managing diet, lifestyle, and stress. Some people with IBS need medication and counseling. IBS can occur at any age, but it often begins in the teen years or in early adulthood. It is twice as common in women as in men.

Inflammatory bowel disease, on the other hand, is more insidious. Crohn's disease and ulcerative colitis are autoimmune disorders that afflict boys and girls, men and women alike at any age, although the most common ages of onset are between 15 and 30 and after 50.

With IBD, the immune system mistakes harmless food, bacteria, and other materials in the intestine for invading or infectious substances. In response, the body sends white blood cells into the lining of the intestines, where they produce chronic inflammation and ulcerations. It is as if an AK-47 had invaded your body to eradicate ladybugs in unpredictable spurts for as long as you lived. (For more details about this reaction of the immune system, you can visit: www.ccfa.org/what-are-crohns-and-colitis/.)

The difference between the symptoms of Crohn's disease and ulcerative colitis can be stark or so subtle that the diagnosis eludes even a gastroenterologist and the usually definitive tests.

About 1.6 million Americans have IBD, with 70,000 new cases diagnosed each year. When the diagnosis is unclear, you may be told you have Crohn's colitis, which doesn't mean you have both diseases, only that you have Crohn's disease located solely in your large intestine. If the diagnosis is "indeterminate" Crohn's colitis, it means that it is unclear whether you have ulcerative colitis or Crohn's disease.

With Crohn's disease, the inflammation can be sporadic, leaving normal areas between patches of diseased intestine. Although the disease usually affects the end of the small intestine and the beginning of the colon, Crohn's can occur anywhere in the digestive tract, from the mouth to the anus, the ulcerations spreading into all layers of the bowel walls. As one mother explained to her 11-year-old son who had just been diagnosed, "Crohn's is like having a canker sore from the tip of your tongue through your digestive tract all the way to your *tush*. Some of the sores are open and sore and bleeding. That's why it hurts so much."

Ulcerative colitis creates continuous areas of inflammation in the lining of the large intestine and rectum. It stops at the juncture of the large and small intestine and goes no higher. The lining develops open tiny sores or ulcers that produce pus, blood, and mucous. Colitis characteristically causes an acute urgency to run to the bathroom, often to expel nothing but pus and blood.

The discomfort and pain that people with IBS grapple with should not be minimized. However, to misunderstand the difference between two strikingly similar-sounding conditions is to create a false comparison between a stress-related illness and an autoimmune disease. People with IBS can reasonably expect to relieve their symptoms with a change of diet, medication, and relaxation techniques. People with IBD would be grateful if that's what it took to banish their incurable illness.

Epidemiology – When and Where IBD Is Found

Sir Samuel Wilks, a 19th-century British physician, first used the term "ulcerative colitis" in a case report in 1859. Crohn's disease was first identified in the 19th century, and the first study was published in 1913. However, the disease didn't get its name until 1932, when Dr. Burrill B. Crohn, an American gastroenterologist, and two colleagues published a paper describing its characteristics.

Perhaps because all 14 patients in Dr. Crohn's original study were Jewish, a misperception formed that IBD is found mostly among Ashkenazic Jews, Jews of Eastern European ancestry. (This misunderstanding delayed the diagnosis of at least one patient, Kevin Anderson, as described in Chapter Three). Since then, there has been a perceived association between Jewish ethnicity and an increased risk of IBD. Although it is true that IBD is two to four times more prevalent among Ashkenazic Jews than among non-Jewish whites, the vast majority of people with IBD are not Jewish. Crohn's and ulcerative colitis are most common in European and North American populations, including African Americans, and least common in Hispanics and Asians, although as environments around the world become more Westernized, it is theorized that IBD will spread to those populations as well.

Further undermining the belief that IBD is a Jewish disease, the rates of IBD in Israel do not differ from those in the United Kingdom and Scandinavia. The author of an epidemiological survey of IBD, Dr. Anders Ekbom of the Karolinska University Hospital in Stockholm, Sweden, concludes, "It is theorized that environmental factors, not genetics with ethnicity, are the major driving force for the increase in incidence over time."

Curiously, researchers found that when the incidence of ulcerative colitis rose in a country they studied, the incidence of Crohn's disease rose 20 years later. Dr. Ekbom theorized that ulcerative colitis and Crohn's disease "represent the opposite ends of a continuous spectrum of one disease entity, but with different clinical characteristics." He also speculated that there "are some shared genetic and/or environmental risk factors for ulcerative colitis and Crohn's disease." (Ekbom, 2004)

Genetic Factors

For those given to brooding over the possibility that a relative might develop IBD, here is a grab bag of statistics. It is important to remember that epidemiology is the study of large populations, not individuals. If someone has a 7-to-9 percent greater chance of developing IBD, they have a

91-to-93 percent chance of *not* developing it.

- There seems to be a stronger risk of inheriting Crohn's disease than ulcerative colitis, especially in families of Jewish descent.
- Children who have one parent with Crohn's disease have a 7-to-9 percent lifetime risk of developing the condition and a 10 percent risk of developing some form of IBD.
- Children of two parents who have IBD have a 35 percent risk of developing some form of IBD.
- Approximately 20 percent of people with IBD have a family member with the disease, and their risk of developing IBD is 10 times higher than for persons in the general population.
- The risk of IBD for persons who have a sibling with IBD is 30 times higher than for persons in the general population. (Tresca, 2015)

Many genes carrying susceptibility for IBD have been identified, with at least 33 of them currently well established for Crohn's disease. It is more difficult to find a specific number of genes associated with ulcerative colitis, because the source of the disease seems more complicated. However, because researchers are making great strides in mapping the genome, a more complete genetic picture of IBD may emerge.

It is believed that for those with a genetic predisposition, IBD develops when a genetically susceptible host is exposed to a series of environmental triggers. These triggers chronically activate the immune system of the intestinal lining, which we recognize clinically as Crohn's disease or ulcerative colitis. However, only 20 percent of people with IBD have the genetics for it. That leaves 80 percent with no apparent genetic connection to the disease and with only environmental factors to blame.

Environmental Triggers

Despite an onslaught of studies trying to identify the environmental factors that cause Crohn's and ulcerative colitis, researchers continually seem to hit a dead end. One of my favorites is the cat correlation. According to a survey published in the *Journal of Gastroenterology and Hepatology*, Crohn's disease patients diagnosed in adulthood were less likely to have lived with a cat before they were 5 years old. However, patients who were more at risk of developing Crohn's in childhood were more likely to live with a cat before age 5. (Amre, 2006) Now, what are parents who own cats supposed to do with this information? Should expectant parents get rid of their cat just to be on the safe side? If scientists could isolate something about cats that connects with IBD and formulate a theory of its cause, that study would have some meaning. Otherwise, it breeds only guilt among parents of children with Crohn's who had a cat when their child was under the age of 5.

Smoking remains the most widely studied and replicated risk factor. But smoking is paradoxical in its effect on IBD. Despite all the harm it does in every area of the body, smoking may confer protection against ulcerative colitis. However, it contributes to an increased risk for and severity of Crohn's disease. (Ashwin, 2013) Nevertheless, I began to smoke when I was 12 (I am not proud of this) and I was diagnosed with ulcerative colitis at 16. (For the record, I quit smoking at 25.) For years, I assumed that I'd helped to bring on my colitis with those cigarettes. So, in my case, while smoking may not have caused my colitis, it certainly didn't confer protection against it, either. As Dr. Ekbom put it succinctly in one presentation, "No, we cannot predict the natural history on an individual level." (Ekbom, 2004)

In short, the evidence of the environment's role in causing the onset of IBD is muddy. "Almost every new chemical compound introduced in a population during the last 100 years has been proposed to be of importance for the etiology in inflammatory bowel disease," writes Dr. Ekbom. "These include toothpaste, chewing gum, fast food, margarine, cornflakes, etc. … The common characteristic of studies on such exposures is that they deal with small patient groups with data assembled retrospectively." (Ekbom, 2006) In short, the studies are full of holes.

But researchers plug on. The findings have real consequences, though not always beneficial ones for families. Each time a new hypothesis is published, anxious parents apply the information to their child with IBD, concerned that this or that aspect of their lifestyle is influencing the degree or frequency of flare-ups of their disease. It doesn't matter that many of the studies involve the cause — not the exacerbation — of IBD. It can be crazy making.

As the authors of Dr. Ekbom's survey sadly conclude, "Despite years of investigation, the environmental risk factors that have been identified have not explained the pathogenesis [the manner of development] of IBD. Several environmental factors, such as smoking, appendicitis, oral contraceptive pills, diet, breastfeeding, infections/vaccinations, antibiotics, helminthes (intestinal parasites), and childhood hygiene have been implicated in the increased worldwide incidence of IBD. However, even the most consistently demonstrated environmental risk factor, smoking, contributes only partially to disease pathogenesis (i.e., most smokers do not have Crohn's disease and most Crohn's patients do not smoke). Thus, further studies are necessary to better understand the environmental determinants of IBD."

CHAPTER THREE
Diagnosis: Delay and Confusion

After spending nearly a decade running to the bathroom with diarrhea several times a day, Adina, a college student, became seriously worried when she began to bleed from her rectum. Away from home, she decided to handle it herself, so she went to a Kaiser medical clinic near her university. She saw a doctor who listened to her symptoms, which included stomach pain and weight loss. The doctor told her that she might have AIDS. "I'm staring at her," she said heatedly as she recounted the scene to me eight years later. "I asked her, 'How can you say that? Have you checked my blood? Couldn't it be stomach flu?' I ran out of there, demanding to see someone else." She immediately called her uncle, a Kaiser executive. He said it sounded as if she had Crohn's disease or ulcerative colitis. Two days later, Adina was properly tested and the ulcerative colitis diagnosis was confirmed.

While this story may seem like an outlier, sad to say, it is not. Adina's story is only slightly unusual because the doctor suggested a more serious illness rather than a less serious cause for her symptoms and because Adina had a connection in the medical world that provided her with a speedy diagnosis. One study found that it takes twice as long to diagnose Crohn's disease than ulcerative colitis — two years, compared with one. (Oliva-Hemker, 2010) But 40 percent of the patients with whom I spoke were sent down dead ends for years before getting a definitive diagnosis of IBD. And few had the personal connections that would have hastened the process.

One of the reasons the path to a diagnosis of IBD is often crooked and rocky is that IBD is not the first thing a pediatrician, a family physician, or even a gastroenterologist may consider when hearing your symptoms. In fact, you may be told that you have one of many other conditions that can be explained by the very same symptoms, among them IBS, flu, bleeding hemorrhoids, gastroenteritis, food poisoning, parasites, anorexia, appendicitis, bad eating habits, anxiety, or depression. Quite an array of diseases has to be ruled out.

"Many of the symptoms of IBD are not specific and could occur in any number of health conditions," write the authors of *Your Child with Inflammatory Bowel Disease: A Family Guide for Caregiving*. "Even pediatric gastroenterologists don't assume that their own child's abdominal pain and diarrhea [mean] he or she has IBD."

The patient accounts I heard highlight the stress that children and parents must bear while symptoms rage and no cause can be found. These stories are intended to let those of you with similar experiences know that you are not alone, that it is not unusual for IBD to be initially missed. These stories also let those of you who were diagnosed fairly quickly understand how fortunate you were to find out what was wrong without delay, even given the difficulties that lay ahead. Finally, the stories will, I hope, encourage families and partners of young people to keep searching for the best ways to support them with patience and equanimity while they search for answers to their symptoms.

Causes for Delays

Besides the similarity of IBD symptoms to other ailments, there are many other reasons for delays in getting to the diagnosis of Crohn's disease or colitis. Let's start with patients who are numbed by fear and who avoid seeking medical attention in the hope that the symptoms will disappear on their own.

Wishful Thinking

The first symptoms of Crohn's and ulcerative colitis may throw you into confusion. You may be paralyzed by seeing blood painlessly filling a toilet bowl or by experiencing sharp stomach pain. Weeks or months can pass before you can bring yourself to speak up. Sometimes, your mind jumps to thoughts of cancer. Your initial impulse is not to alarm those closest to you, particularly your parents. Hope battles reason. The hope persists: Maybe it will go away. So you don't say anything for a while, sometimes a long while.

LoriAnn is one such person. She was rarely sick until she was 20, when she dropped 25 pounds in a month. She endured nausea, rectal bleeding, and cramping, but she felt that she should be able to handle it herself. So she said nothing to her mother and went alone to see her family doctor. When LoriAnn compared the symptoms to her idea of what morning sickness must be like, the doctor ventured, "Well, girls your age are getting pregnant. Why don't you take a pregnancy test?" She felt dispirited. She was only using morning sickness as an illustration. She knew she wasn't pregnant. "I didn't know where to go," she told me. "My family didn't know about it. I was scared out of my mind." So she did nothing. Two months had passed when Lori saw a TV ad sponsored by the Crohn's and Colitis Foundation of America (CCFA) and learned a new word: gastroenterologist. She found one on the Internet and went to see him by herself. She finally told her mother what was going on only when she needed a ride home after being anesthetized for a colonoscopy. The test diagnosed her ulcerative colitis, resolving months of isolation and confusion.

Doctors on the Wrong Path

While patients unwittingly delay the diagnosis because they deny that their symptoms are serious, physicians may unknowingly take families down the wrong path when warning signs are flashing.

A mother who had a hunch about her son's symptoms ran into resistance from his pediatrician. Cathy's 11-year-old son, David, began suffering stomach cramps and he could barely eat. She took him to his pediatrician, who speculated that a parasite going around might be responsible. "Could it be Crohn's disease?" Cathy asked her, because she had a good friend whose daughter had Crohn's and it sounded like her son's symptoms. "Don't be so histrionic," the pediatrician replied, curtly dismissing her concern. Cathy wasn't deterred. A physician friend quickly got David in to see a gastroenterologist at the Children's Hospital of Philadelphia, who made an immediate diagnosis of Crohn's disease. The entire process — from first symptoms to diagnosis — took four weeks.

Many patients and families aren't so lucky. It took family connections to get that appointment, just as it did with Adina. Not everyone has the luxury of knowing a doctor who is friendly with a top-notch gastroenterologist. It also took a parent who refused to take no for an answer and who followed her own instincts.

Jacque, who was living on a U.S. Air Force base in Idaho, initially did not follow her instincts, so she accepted her doctor's reassurance that her toddler, Josh, would be all right, given time. At 18 months, Josh had developed rashes, boils, and fistulas (an infected tunnel under the skin near the rectum). His bowels were loose and he was extremely lethargic. Jacque thought she would lose him. The pediatrician admitted Josh to the hospital, where he still wasn't thriving after a week. Nevertheless, the doctor dismissed her concerns. "He'll always be a loose-bowel kid," he told Jacque. "He'll be fine by age 5." He wasn't.

At 5 ½, Josh had an accident in his pants in kindergarten, and he later lost control at three pool parties. Jacque was going through a divorce at the time, and she thought that the incidents, horrible and embarrassing as they were, might be due to stress. She moved with Josh back to her home state of Delaware, where Josh was still, in her words, "a helpless kid who couldn't walk without losing control of his bowels. He was a sick little boy."

At her wit's end, she took Josh to another doctor, who didn't think the divorce was causing his problems. He referred them to the Nemours/Alfred I. DuPont Hospital for Children in Wilmington, Delaware, where she was told to prepare Josh for a colonoscopy and an endoscopy. The tests were conclusive. Josh had Crohn's disease and, after hearing his history, the gastroenterologist said that he'd probably been living with it since he was 18 months old.

Rural vs. Urban

Other issues, too, get in the way of a speedy diagnosis. Compassion and skill know no geographical boundaries, but certainly large urban teaching hospitals see many more IBD patients than do smaller hospitals. So, while many patients live near a major medical center, many others go to local hospitals, where doctors are less likely to identify the obvious signs of IBD.

Jessica, who was 17 when we spoke, began feeling sick in the eighth grade. Five times she was taken to the emergency room in the hospital up the street. "They just kept saying, 'Try this, try that,'" she recalled. "Nothing worked." She was down to 93 pounds. Her pediatrician thought she had anorexia. Her family ultimately took her to a larger, regional hospital where a doctor performed the necessary tests and diagnosed her with Crohn's disease two years after her symptoms began.

It took longer than five years and numerous doctors' visits before Trinity was diagnosed with ulcerative colitis at age 8. Trinity's anatomy had been sending out signals since she was 18 months old, but, after all, ulcerative colitis is not the first thing that physicians think about when they see a toddler in distress. Instead, the doctors in the local hospital in Bethlehem, Pennsylvania kept treating her symptoms.

At age 2, Trinity complained of joint pain, which a doctor attributed to growing pains. At age 3, Trinity couldn't urinate because her urinary tract was blocked. Her doctor said she had more stool inside her than the average adult male, and he gave her a stool softener. At age 7, ulcers on her scalp, arms, legs, and abdomen "almost looked to my husband and me as if we had burned her with cigarettes," remembered her mother, LeAnne. The family doctor said it must be eczema, but a dermatologist couldn't diagnose her condition. Then, a day after her eighth birthday, Trinity came home and told LeAnne she didn't feel well. She said there was blood in the toilet.

LeAnne didn't panic. Sometimes, she thought, kids strain and get a fissure, a tear in the rectum that can bleed. "We started dinner and she starts screaming bloody murder in the bathroom and when I run in, my exact words are 'holy s—-.' It looks like she'd gotten her period."

Even this serious development didn't lead to a diagnosis. After being seen at a local hospital, Trinity was sent home with antibiotics. During the next two months, as Trinity became sicker and sicker, her mother tried to get an appointment with a gastroenterologist, but no one could see her for weeks. She took Trinity to a regional hospital, where she was admitted and, for two weeks, was tested for parasites and every ailment but IBD. Trinity hated to eat, because food sent her to the bathroom where she would bleed, so she drank only chicken broth. The hospital inserted an intravenous line to get nutrition directly into her body.

Finally, physicians decided to perform a colonoscopy. Only a few minutes into the procedure, the doctor came out and told her parents that Trinity had ulcerative colitis. LeAnne had never heard of it. She showed the gastroenterologist photographs of Trinity's old skin condition and told him about her other symptoms. The doctor told her that ulcerative colitis was associated with all her symptoms, but until the diagnosis was made, the connections were missed.

Financial Issues

Then there is the financial consideration. Many patients have medical insurance and can afford to have their symptoms thoroughly investigated, because the hospital and physicians can expect some compensation from insurance companies. However, many patients do not have insurance, although under the Affordable Care Act, it is hoped, those numbers will shrink.

Kevin, a native of Lafayette, Louisiana, whose symptoms began when he was a high school sophomore, suffered a double whammy: He didn't fit the perceived profile of someone with Crohn's disease and, growing up poor, he had no health insurance. Multiple times after suffering severe cramps, he went to the University Medical Center emergency room, but the doctors there sent him home each time, saying he had gas. They told him to take Mylanta for indigestion. "I took so much Mylanta that when I'm in a drugstore even now and see Mylanta bottles, I want to throw up," Kevin said years later.

On yet another visit to the emergency room, a physician looked at his x-rays and told Kevin that a pocket of air was causing his pain. "I couldn't take it any more," Kevin recollected. "I got down on my hands and knees and begged the doctor to cut me open. I wrapped my arms around his knees and wouldn't let go until he agreed to do surgery." The physician complied. During exploratory surgery, doctors found that Kevin had a complete bowel obstruction. Had they sent him home again, there was a strong possibility that he would have died.

At one point, Kevin overheard a discussion between two doctors about his case. "They weren't familiar with Crohn's disease at all around here in southern Louisiana in the early '90s," he told me. "But one surgeon was a guy from New York, and he talked about me having Crohn's disease. The other doctor said no way possible, because I was black and I was male and Crohn's was just found in Jewish white women. The New York doctor tried to explain to him that Crohn's could be diagnosed in anyone."

Kevin's quest didn't end there. It took several more visits to the emergency room before the gastroenterologist finally relented and performed the colonoscopy that diagnosed him with Crohn's disease.

These cases illustrate the breakdowns that can occur when doctors look at a set of symptoms rather than listening carefully to a patient's story and keeping an open mind.

Avoidance

Another impediment to a smooth diagnosis occurs when you hear what the doctor is saying, but don't really take it in.

Joel was old enough to understand the meaning of the word "chronic" when his physician used it to diagnose him with ulcerative colitis. Even so, complained Joel, when he was 28, "I didn't know what chronic meant. This doctor diagnosed what's going to be with me forever after a two-minute conversation. I was so angry at how he handled it." Still somewhat in shock, Joel expected that his illness would resolve itself like every other time he had been sick and gotten better when he took cold medicine or an antibiotic. And although he was warned by the doctor not to believe everything he read on the Internet about ulcerative colitis, he went straight to his computer anyway. "That's where I found out that 'chronic' meant this is with you forever," Joel said.

The full implications of the word "chronic" also eluded Alisa when she was diagnosed at age 22. The doctor gave her a pamphlet and a prescription and asked if she had any questions. "Umm, yes, my main question is, what the — — is going on?" she recalled. "Actually, I wasn't super alarmed. I was just happy to have a diagnosis and a way to treat it. Seemed like a one-two punch. One, you have colitis. Two, take this drug and it will go away." Alisa didn't remember her doctor explaining that the disease would not go away. "The doctor may have told me that, but I'm fairly sure something like that would stick in my head," she said nine years after her diagnosis. She remembered that the thrust of his message was "not to worry, don't change a thing, just take these pills and you'll be fine."

Looking back, Alisa admitted that she didn't want to know how intractable IBD would be. "The fact that he made it no big deal was almost better," she said, but she wished that he had more fully explained, "that this would be a long-term situation, that it would not go away and that the disease needed to be addressed on many different levels. If I had understood the depth of what it was," she said, "I would have approached it differently."

Alisa's ambivalence is very human. On being diagnosed, you certainly want to know what's wrong, but you may not be ready to hear the whole story. You may blame the physician as the bearer of bad news and yet also fault the physician for not delivering all the bad news.

The Tests

Your first step toward a diagnosis occurs when you provide a stool sample, an act that goes against every cultural norm. As I discussed in the introduction, the repugnance when dealing with your stool's look and smell is culturally universal (although, somehow, dog owners do manage to pick up their dogs' stool without feeling repulsion every time. Don't we love ourselves as much as we love our dogs?)

Joel expressed revulsion when his doctor asked him to get a stool sample after hearing that he had experienced acute symptoms after eating an oatmeal cookie and that he had diarrhea whenever he ate anything. His internist said it was probably food poisoning. Joel's recollection of collecting those samples vividly describes what many patients face. "There was a pungent smell, especially because I wasn't having solid stools," he recalled in the sonorous voice he used in his work as a health and wellness coach and yoga teacher. "I had to put this plastic spoon into my stool to move it into this container. It was highly disgusting and gross. Then I walked into the office holding my poop. I gave it to the woman at the counter, trying to keep a straight face."

If the stool sample comes up negative for other ailments, the tests can be as difficult and demeaning as the disease itself. No matter which tests are performed, they invade your private body parts in ways that induce feelings of submission and even humiliation. Thus do sigmoidoscopies, endoscopies and colonoscopies introduce you to your future: uncomfortable, painful symptoms leading to uncomfortable and undignified tests to track the course of your uncomfortable, embarrassing, and painful disease.

Josh was 6 when his mother, Jacque, had to prepare him for his first colonoscopy. Jacque recalled the scene. "'I have to put a quart of this in your little hiney,' which wasn't big enough to fit the whole quart in. He looked up at me and said, 'I'm sorry I'm sick. I'm sorry you have to do this to me.' Then he leaned over the side of the tub."

As rarely as colonoscopies are administered to 6 year olds, there are legitimate reasons why the three major tests for IBD are not more readily administered to patients of any age. These are the tests of last resort. They are expensive and invasive, and they often require anesthesia, which is why they are not performed at the drop of a hat. The physician has to strongly suspect IBD in order to justify ordering them.

"In some cases, the symptoms and signs are very subtle and we or the families are reluctant to put the kids through invasive studies (endoscopy) or radiologic studies," said Dr. Keith Benkov, associate professor of pediatric gastroenterology at Mount Sinai hospital in New York City and former head of the department. "We like to make as early a diagnosis as possible, as we think early treatment is preventative. [But] sometimes when we do our studies too early, there are not enough findings to make a firm diagnosis. Though studies are invasive, they are easily and safely accomplished with our newer techniques."

When your doctor gets past other possibilities and decides that the test is justified, you must brace yourself physically and emotionally for the bodily invasion. Perhaps the most difficult aspect of undergoing these procedures is the feeling of disassociation that is required to get through them. The best and perhaps only thing to do is to detach yourself from what is happening to your body and maintain some modicum of dignity.

A sigmoidoscopy requires you to lie on your side on the examining table, knees to chest. Perhaps your eyes are closed; perhaps you are staring into space or at the bookcase across the room. The doctor is out of sight behind you and temporarily out of relationship with you. The sigmoidoscope he pushes into your rectum will view the inside of your descending colon by pumping air into the large intestine to make the tissue inside visible. As Joel described it, the doctor performing his sigmoidoscopy "was blowing up a balloon and the balloon was my colon." If there are ulcerations in the descending colon, this test will see them. You will probably want to shower after this test, to cleanse yourself of the lubricant and your feelings that went with it.

Another test commonly given to diagnose Crohn's disease (and other gastrointestinal illnesses as well) is an upper G.I. series, in which you drink a chalky concoction of x-ray-sensitive barium. With the affected area illuminated by the barium, a doctor inserts a tube into your mouth and threads it down your esophagus into the upper gastrointestinal tract. You are usually sedated enough so that you do not gag. Patients' accounts of undergoing an upper G.I. series run the gamut from horrific to no big deal, especially when sedation is involved. Drinking the barium is universally reviled. "He had to drink the barium, which is extremely hard for a 9 year old," Hillary said of her son Jordan. "He was throwing it up. The colonoscopy was a lot easier."

That may have been the first time the words "easier" and "colonoscopy" were included in the same sentence during my interviews. A colonoscopy is a definitive test for both Crohn's disease and ulcerative colitis. You are sedated to the point of unconsciousness or extreme grogginess. A long flexible tube is inserted into your rectum. The tube snakes all the way up through the large intestine — where ulcerative colitis occurs in continuous stretches — to the juncture of the small intestine. It may then rise into the terminal ileum, at the end of the small intestine, where Crohn's often appears in discontinuous patches.

The most challenging part of the colonoscopy is the preparation, which involves emptying the entire colon of stool. Younger children and teenagers, who must drink large quantities of laxative and who must clutch the contents of an enema until they can't hold it in anymore, will do it because their parents tell them they must. The rest of us do it because, well, we understand the imperative to clean out our colon for the test.

Now that people over 50 are advised to undergo a colonoscopy to screen for colon cancer, the test has become more ubiquitous. Healthy people now have to prepare for the test every five or ten years. They have to confront what I went through every year, which made Dave Barry's account of his preparation for a colonoscopy all the more hilarious to me.

Barry, a humorist and newspaper columnist, wrote: "In accordance with my instructions, I didn't eat any solid food that day; all I had was chicken broth, which is basically water, only with less flavor. Then, in the evening, I took the MoviPrep. You mix two packets of powder together in a one-liter plastic jug, and then you fill it with lukewarm water. (For those unfamiliar with the metric system, a liter is about 32 gallons.) Then you have to drink the whole jug. This takes about an hour, because MoviPrep tastes — and here I am being kind — like a mixture of goat spit and urinal cleanser, with just a hint of lemon."

Dahlia expressed what most patients would say after undergoing any of these tests. They "made me feel sicker. That's what I remember. All the tests were incredibly unpleasant. There's got to be a way to diagnose without making a patient so miserable."

Indeed, procedures that may be only mildly unpleasant to people without IBD, can truly distress people with IBD in the short term. For example, I bled more heavily for days and experienced more severe cramping after a sigmoidoscopy or colonoscopy, largely because when you insert any instrument into already ulcerated tissue, the tissue will become even more reactive. So, administering the tests has a reward/risk aspect to it. The intrusion of a tube into an already sensitive and inflamed colon or small intestine has to be withstood, but the collateral damage also has to be endured.

Unfortunately, to date, there just is no innocuous way to diagnose IBD. Once the diagnosis is made, you will certainly want a full accounting of the physical challenges you will likely confront, if you're ready to take them in. You will also want your doctor to understand the emotional and social implications that IBD will impose on your life. If your doctor is unable to provide this psychological support or even to acknowledge the necessity of such support, it would be helpful if he or she refers you to a professional who is familiar with the issues that chronic disease can impose and with your need to learn self-compassion and patience.

CHAPTER FOUR

Responding to the Diagnosis

At first, patients and their families feel their dispiriting burden somewhat lightened when a diagnosis finally provides a name to what has long afflicted them.

At the hospital, when doctors told Charlotte that she had Crohn's disease, she felt improbably happy. "Relieved. I wasn't crazy. It was something that was real and I could treat it," she told me. Before her diagnosis at age 14, after five years of symptoms, Charlotte was "very depressed when I had all my symptoms and I didn't know what was wrong."

When Adina was finally diagnosed after almost a decade of symptoms, her parents understood at last why their daughter kept asking them to stop the car on road trips so she could run to the bathroom. They used to tell her, "You're a big girl. You can wait." But after the diagnosis, they knew that she couldn't, because she had ulcerative colitis.

Gratitude would seem an unlikely emotion when you're diagnosed with IBD, but that's just what Dahlia felt on learning, at 17, that she had Crohn's disease. "My response was, this could have been cancer. I'm very fortunate. This is treatable. My other response was, 50 years earlier, I would have died without modern medicine. I came away from it with appreciation, feeling fortunate that it was treatable."

When undiagnosed symptoms have stopped you from doing what you love to do, you can move on with your life after you learn what's wrong. Chelsea, 28, was diagnosed with Crohn's disease at age 13. "The diagnosis — figuring out what was wrong with me — consumed so much of my life," she recalled. "I was a big soccer player. I danced and did all the shows in school. All of that was on hold. Going through all the tests was the hardest part. Once I started feeling better, I didn't want it to become who I was. It was something I just deal with." She became an actress and a singer who understudied the title role in "The Little Mermaid" on Broadway and played the title role on the road.

After the diagnosis, patients and families have to tackle a cascade of challenges. The first, of course, is to obtain adequate medical treatment. Another is to learn effective self-care, to investigate what works and what doesn't alleviate your particular symptoms. But perhaps your most ambitious undertaking is to move socially and emotionally toward self-acceptance. As Chelsea noted, you don't want to allow the disease to define you.

Besides feeling the positive emotions when young people grasp that they have a new, unwelcome companion for life, newly diagnosed patients also encounter a sweeping fear of the unknown.

Emmett, a 22-year-old drummer, was diagnosed at the end of freshman year of high school, after six months of such crippling, paralytic pain that he would become nauseated whenever he ate. He became anemic and rapidly lost weight. "I didn't know what was happening. I didn't know if I would die. I was in complete darkness," he said. "That put me in a horrible, horrible place." He noted that before the diagnosis, "something's going wrong and we don't know what it is. Afterwards, we know there's this thing I have, but there's no cure and no effective treatment. Everyone's different and I have to figure it out."

Adam acknowledges and accepts the unknowns about his disease. "One thing I've learned is how little doctors understand the process of Crohn's. There's a lot of genetic machinery associated with it, but in terms of the mechanisms involved, there's still a lot to learn and it's manifested in my treatment. I've tried drugs to no effect. They're cobbling their story together," he said of his doctors. "They frequently don't really know what's going on. Why are you having a flare-up? Why do I not have urgency when a lot of other people do? Why can I eat some things and not others, and why do other people react differently? We have to assign doctors a great deal of knowledge, and often they know incredible things, but they take on an aura of supreme knowledge, which they really don't have about these things. It's a very slow process of accumulating knowledge, and we often don't know what's going on. They don't even know why these diseases are autoimmune disorders."

Creating a Bond with Your GI Doc

Despite the many difficult stories about doctors who take patients down dead-end paths, close, positive relationships between doctors and patients can and do occur. Many patients have satisfying relationships with their physicians, a few of whom even have Crohn's or colitis themselves and who know firsthand the full impact that the diagnosis will impose on patients and families.

Many young patients, in fact, become so attached to their pediatric gastroenterologists that when they age out of pediatrics, it is a devastating loss. As with a first love, you never forget your first gastroenterologist.

Jill, who was diagnosed with Crohn's at age 7, was a graduate student at Tufts University researching the social aspects of IBD when she spoke about the transition to adult care from pediatrics. She had a rough transition. "You're used to one doctor and then you get what they call a "big kid GI." They just treat you differently. It's not as warm and fuzzy. When you've been in peds (pediatrics) for 15 years and all of a sudden you're not in peds, you say to yourself, 'I can do this.' Then you get there, and you're like, 'It's scary.' You're there by yourself. Your parents aren't there anymore. In undergrad, I still went home to my pediatric appointments, but I live a long way from home now and my parents aren't going to fly up for a doctor's appointment."

Karen finally had to leave her pediatric GI doctor when she was 21 and a senior in college, after she was told she needed an adult doctor. "Every time I went to the children's hospital, they would look for a baby and I'd say, 'No, it's me.' I was pushing it for sure," she acknowledged, adding, "I don't get the same attention, understanding, or quality of care I got from my pediatric guy."

"Those transitions from a children's hospital, which is warmer and with many more people to interface with, to adult physicians who are much more distant — it's a huge transition, huge," said Dr. Christine Kodman-Jones, a psychologist who used to work in the GI department of a children's hospital. "You feel like you're a part of a mill more than a clinic designed to support you. I think that's the reality. There used to be a program to help kids transition to an adult G.I. doc. The world of medicine is a tough one. If you want information, you have to work it yourself."

Unfortunately, many of the patients and families interviewed indicated that warm, fuzzy relationships, even with pediatric gastroenterologists, occur more rarely than more impersonal ones. A physician enumerates the reasons for this.

"I think that, as physicians, we don't know what it feels like to be patients or to have certain types of illnesses," said a GI doc who asked not to be identified. "A doctor needs to be functional. We're very matter-of-fact about surgery, tests, and hospitals. But, as physicians, we're not trained to say how we would feel if a family member were a patient and how unpleasant it is. I don't think [doctors] slow down and think about it. I've seen lots of [doctors] be very matter of fact about it. Physicians who do better are those who can empathize."

It has always struck me as heroic that some physicians choose to specialize in Crohn's disease and colitis at all, knowing that their patients will never be cured, at least in the foreseeable future. In dealing with intractable diseases, each physician has a daily challenge to open his or her heart again and again. Some do. Some do not.

Many physicians are uncomfortable entering nonlinear territory, especially the psychological impact on IBD patients and their families. Dealing with patients' emotional upset and stress takes them outside the realm of their medical training. Although not every doctor is naturally adept with a human touch, many can establish a rapport with parents and children.

"In pediatrics, we have to establish rapport with both the parents and the child, especially in adolescence," Dr. Benkov observed. "For parents, we have to show that we are knowledgeable and experienced but willing to listen to what they have to say and have a dialogue. We have to make sure they have time to express themselves, both to us and sometimes our other staff. Even connecting different families can be helpful. It is also helpful when we can easily demonstrate that we easily remember small details of both their medical cases and outside information. For the kids it is relatively easy in terms of just showing that we care and are interested in them - which sounds simple but you cannot fake anything with kids. Sometimes kids who are going through a lot of emotional issues, as well as parents, are hard to get through to and often need a team approach."

Patients notice when doctors are able to connect and when they are not. "I think it's important to find a doctor you're comfortable with," said Michal of Boston, who was diagnosed in her early 20s. "I found top G.I. doctors in Philadelphia, Boston, and Israel, and I found them to be very pompous. They're well known, at the top of their field, but I didn't feel seen as a person, but just a medical case. I felt it was hard to find a doctor who was personable, who clearly knows what they're doing, and someone I feel comfortable with."

Perhaps doctors find it necessary to harden their hearts. Otherwise, they could become swallowed up in their patients' misery. It is a technique that psychologists learn, to empathize without absorbing their patients' unhappiness.

Also, time with the doctor is short and there is little opportunity to talk. Jill has worked to devise a pre-appointment visit plan to help young people get their points across in the doctor's office. She believes that young people could use email and texts to help them better communicate with their physicians without taking up precious time in the office.

"You go into the [doctor's office] for fifteen minutes," she said. "You have five or six important points you want to discuss. Pediatric patients freeze when they go into the office. You feel rushed. It's not anyone's fault. It's the system."

A Doctor-Patient Fantasy

I heard so many stories about unsatisfactory IBD appointments in physicians' offices that an image began to form about how an ideal doctor-patient relationship would address patients' concerns when the diagnosis is handed down.

How gratifying it would be for a physician to sit down with a young patient or parent, take their hands, and explain the full story of IBD. This is what such a doctor might say to you:

"Okay, you will probably experience pain and discomfort. The medications will help, but maybe not always and maybe not forever. This disease poses a challenge, both physically and emotionally. It may be difficult for you to talk about it with your friends. You may need to run to the bathroom and interrupt playing sports or a date or a movie. You may be too embarrassed to talk about why you have to leave, but I urge you to talk about your IBD to everyone you trust. It's important that you do so, because it will help you to accept this fact about yourself, that you have a chronic illness that feels embarrassing and that until now cannot be cured.

"Going forward, you have a choice. You can be debilitated and victimized by your condition. Or you can become emotionally stronger by dealing with this disease. You may mature more quickly, because IBD can make you more compassionate and empathetic toward others. You will understand what it means to have a difficult condition that you played no role in developing and that won't go away. Let me repeat this: You had no role in developing this disease. And it won't go away. That is what 'chronic' means. To date, we have no cure. You will understand what it means to be trapped by circumstances beyond your control.

"And I will probably be seeing a lot of you. So let's begin a good relationship. I can refer you to a social worker or psychologist on staff who can answer many of your questions, but I'll be available when you need me."

Finally, your physician in this fictional monologue would tell you about the treatment he or she will prescribe, with all the pros and cons. And your physician will assure you that if or when the medication is no longer effective, there will be others. Your medical treatment is the hurdle to overcome, so you will feel calmer by having someone you trust to guide you.

Back in the real world, few if any doctors react consummately well in every situation. The best you can do when you feel emotionally short-changed is to speak up, without rancor, and tell your physician that you would feel better if he or she would empathize with your struggles or verbally celebrate when your condition improves. It doesn't take more than a moment for a physician to warmly reach out. When patients feel they are in the hands of a human being who can relate to their difficulties, the payoff is incalculable.

In conclusion, with a disease as complex as IBD, it is insufficient for a gastroenterologist to simply conduct a physical exam and write a prescription. Doctors are healers, and healing takes place on many levels, not just physical. It would be helpful for patients if even during their brief, allotted time together, doctors would somehow return to the spirit of Norman Rockwell's painting of a physician who treats both the emotional and physical life of his young patient by putting his stethoscope up to the little girl's doll.

A similar painting done 30 years later, however, would depict a little boy checking the doctor's medical certificate on the wall before getting a shot in his rear, acknowledging that our relationship with physicians has become more distant and more detached. Perhaps physicians and patients together, at least in spirit, can turn the clock back.

CHAPTER FIVE
Coping with Medication

There are remedies, they explained. There are medicines. All I had to do was take seventeen pills a day. Seventeen! And you should've seen these pills! They were horse pills! I could barely choke one down, let alone seventeen a day! I can't even protest because the doctors and my parents and seemingly everyone else in my world are telling me that what I have is very serious and that I have to do everything I can to remedy the damage already done to my colon. That medicine you take, those strong pills of yours, they have side effects. If you don't get your blood tested every six months, you could develop some horrible side effect from the pills you're taking. You could become anemic. How about that!

— A Recluse's Guide
by Ben Brandfon (unpublished novel)

Whether you're trying to conquer your fear of choking on a huge pill or coping with the side effects of drugs that change your appearance and your moods, the art of navigating your medication is a visceral, emotional aspect of coping with IBD. Dealing with your medications and their capricious side effects is part of the process of creating internal stability in the face of external tumult.

Some problems caused by medications can render one almost as socially awkward as IBD itself. You have to remove yourself from friends and daily activities to take your pills or your daily enema, or to get your infusion of medication. If you happen to be someone who doesn't talk about your IBD, you expend a lot of psychic energy to keep your treatment secret. Just the act of taking the medication represents a daily reminder of something you would rather forget — that IBD has a hold on your life and that it will likely flare up without being chronically suppressed by medication.

Some medications require submission and patience. A pill may be too big for your small throat. A steroid enema inserted into your rear will require you to hold the liquid inside of you for as long as possible while the cortisone works on your inflamed rectum. When your parent insists that you take your IBD medication and makes sure you do so, you may feel controlled or intruded upon, and a power struggle may ensue.

Some children are unprepared to swallow large pills. Some adolescents dump their pills, whether out of rebelliousness, resentment, or fear. Image-conscious children and teenagers have to show up at school with distended cheeks and mood swings beyond their capability to control. Young people must figure out how to study and work while remembering to take their medication several times every day.

Since 1990, the pharmaceutical arsenal against IBD has exploded with new medicinal weapons. The oldest medicines still in widespread use are Azulfadine, a sulfa drug introduced in 1949, and Prednisone, a corticosteroid used to suppress the immune system that was approved a year later. Today, shelves are full of medications intended to deal with inflammation and address the underlying causes of symptoms.

Kim said her family was naïve about what they were getting into after her 6-year-old daughter, Chloe, was diagnosed with ulcerative colitis. Kim has another child with juvenile diabetes, which she considers easier to control.

"There's one solution. You take insulin," she said. "Even celiac disease seems simple. You just cut gluten out of your diet." With IBD, though, she tried many medicines for Chloe that were ineffective. "If this one works, you stay with it," she says. "If not, you go to plan B and you keep cycling through these different medications with the expectation that they're not all going to work."

Tracy, who works in the medical field, thought that she could help her teenaged daughter, Lauren, who was diagnosed at 17 with ulcerative colitis. But she found herself unprepared for the unpredictability of the disease and the effects of the medications. "I knew this involved frequent invasive and embarrassing testing for her and medications that would change her lifestyle," Tracy said as she sat next to her daughter in a New Jersey diner. "I didn't know how severely that would happen. I've experienced patients who are put on medication and respond, but when she didn't respond to treatment, it became more and more frustrating. We think she'll take a pill and she'll feel better. When you take a fistful of pills and you don't feel better, it's frustrating."

Let's put effectiveness aside for a moment and look at the sheer volume and size of the pills that some young people with IBD must take.

Scott, 25, who was diagnosed at age 12, said he had to plow through his fear of choking on the large pills he was told to swallow. "Nobody was able to help me get over my fear of choking," he said. "Now I'm a pro. But at first I would not let a pill go past a certain point in my mouth."

At one point, another patient, Louie, was taking 36 pills a day. "You have to carry a big box of pills with you," he said. "It's difficult when you're in a relationship. People get scared and think it's a death sentence." In other words, because of the cocktail of pills he took, people thought that Louie, who is gay, had AIDS.

Rebellion

The long-range implications of IBD may take years for children and adolescents, who tend to feel immortal, to comprehend. One possible response to being overwhelmed by having an incurable disease like IBD is to delude yourself that this isn't really happening and to balk at taking your prescribed medications.

David was diagnosed with Crohn's disease at age 11. He was too young to take giant capsules, so his father would empty his Pentasa into applesauce four times a day. Like everyone else in middle school taking medication, David was supposed to take it in front of the school nurse. But David would go long stretches without showing up at the nurse's office. "I tried to avoid acknowledging that I had something wrong with me," he said. "When I would go for weeks or months without showing up for pills, they would call my dad and he would talk to me about it." Confirming the capriciousness of IBD, his condition remained stable, which convinced young David that the pills were unnecessary.

As he transitioned into high school and greater independence, he staged what he calls his huge rebellion. David's father would put his pills on the kitchen table and David would throw them away when he wasn't looking. His parents didn't discover this until close to the end of his freshman year. They asked David's doctor to tell him why it was so important for him to take his medication. The doctor did that and referred David to a hospital psychologist.

"I don't know what it was within me," said David, who was 26 when we spoke. "Realistically, when people are 16, they take their drugs. It would have been just as easy to take them as to throw them out. Looking back, it was a huge waste of money, something I know about, because now *I'm* paying the bills for my pills. I just didn't want to." And then he got to the heart of his motivation. "I didn't want to show the pain going on inside of me. I was rejecting the idea that Crohn's affected me." In his 20s, David confronted Crohn's full force, as the disease flared so badly that the big-gun medications were summoned to tame it. He has since developed a healthy respect for the power of his disease.

Emma, who was diagnosed at 12, also went through a period of throwing her pills away. Today, as a woman of 30, she attributes her actions to fear. "The whole Crohn's experience was scary and terrifying," she said. "I was supposedly on a high dose of Prednisone and I knew they were slowly increasing the dose. I was afraid I would get sick if they put me on more medicine." By not taking her pills, she became increasingly sick anyway and lost weight. Her doctor, unaware of what was really going on, kept trying a variety of different medications, thinking each was ineffective.

Her physician ultimately realized what was happening. He told Emma's parents that he would have to admit her to the hospital so that the Prednisone could be administered by an intravenous drip. To avoid being hospitalized, Emma confessed. Her parents sent her to a psychiatrist, who suggested that she was trying to get back at her parents, which Emma didn't think was true. "I felt he was trying to put words in my mouth, so I didn't want to see him anymore," she said. Her parents relented, but monitored her medication intake. This led to conflict.

To help her gain weight again, Emma's doctor prescribed a feeding tube in order to give her nutrients that could be absorbed by her body. It was to be threaded down her nose into her stomach every night and taken out each morning. The process of insertion and removal was traumatic. Her father oversaw the whole process. "He would just sit there and I'd refuse to do it for hours," she said. So, her father would wait patiently until Emma was ready.

Emma's mother, a psychologist, "would be hovering in the room, anxious, crying and yelling at me," Emma recalled. Emma sometimes vomited when the tube was pulled out in the morning. Her parents ultimately struck a deal with her. If it took less than half an hour to insert the tube for six nights in a row, she could have the seventh night off. Eventually, the medications kicked in and five months of tube feeding helped her to gain weight. Ironically, all the turmoil over the feeding tube made taking her medications much easier. Emma soon understood the consequences of skipping her medicines. She ground up the pills, put them in her food, and swallowed them.

Rebellion isn't confined to the very young. When a drug you've been taking stops working, frustration can roll into obstinacy. Medicinal enemas worked like a miracle for Alisa, now 25, for a while. She saw the blood "literally switch off overnight. The enemas would go in and I could feel the entire infected part of my colon cool off while the medicine spread through like a welcome breeze."

The enemas worked so well, she was lulled into thinking they had cured her. "Here it was, the reset button I needed to have the colitis go away, have my body be happy once again and I could start fresh," she wrote in her blog, Tiny Little Ulcers. Her euphoria lasted a couple of months.

Like the other drugs Alisa took, the enemas stopped working. "Colitis found a way to keep coming back and tapping me on the shoulder. 'I'm here!' it would say. 'Pay attention to me! I'm telling you to pay attention!' But I didn't get that message. All I thought was that these stupid pills and enemas are not working. I'm not going to take them anymore.'"

So she stopped taking all her medication. "I was in a serious state of denial," she said. "I didn't talk to anyone about it. I just pooped out blood every day and went about my business like it was no big deal. Every few years, I would think to myself, 'Man, I should really get this under control and go back on meds.' I would then take some enemas or pills. The symptoms would clear for a few weeks to a few months and then the blood would come back. I'd get frustrated and go off the pills, then the cycle starts over."

The Emotional Effects of Side Effects

Most drugs prescribed for IBD work capably some of the time, sometimes for a long time, but all have side effects. Prednisone, for example, can be dramatically effective in stemming stubborn symptoms of IBD, but it is notorious for side effects that can wreak havoc on your self-confidence and positive self-image. It creates distended cheeks, sometimes known as chipmunk cheeks or moon face. It causes rapid weight gain in the short term and weakened bones in the long term. It can cause acne to spring up all over your body, just the thing to target you for teasing or bullying. It can cause inexplicable mood swings, causing patients to cry or explode over nothing. It works like a miracle, drying up bleeding and banishing cramps, but Prednisone, even though it brings relief from severe symptoms, creates the worst of times emotionally and socially.

David, now a rabbi in the Midwest, was put on Prednisone for much of his freshman year of college. "The side effects are the worst possible when you're trying to meet girls," he recalled. "I'm sure it was worse in my mind than in reality. I gained weight, my face got puffy, I got acne, all that stuff. You're 18. You're at the peak of your virility. You want to meet girls and go to parties and that wasn't happening."

Doctors usually try to get rampant symptoms under control and then wean patients off Prednisone, prescribing less potent drugs to maintain remission. But a number of people interviewed were unsuccessful in getting off Prednisone. They stayed on much longer than was generally advisable because their symptoms returned every time they were taken off. This led to unintended consequences, both socially and emotionally as well as physically.

Scott was on the drug for nearly a decade. Back in high school, he felt carefree because he was symptom free, thanks to Prednisone. "But it came with consequences," he said five years later. "It made me starving in a way nobody could understand. I had the big puffy cheeks. It made me mad. I was hungry and grumpy." As soon as the dose was reduced, his symptoms would return. He felt chained to the drug. "I knew I shouldn't be on it long term."

But, in making a choice of immediate relief from symptoms over taking seriously the warnings of long-term after-effects, he would say to his parents, "I don't care if it means a bunch of problems now or bigger problems ten years from now. I just want to be on it." A few months before our interview, Scott was taken off Prednisone completely for the first time in almost 10 years and he encountered the repercussions he'd been warned about. "All the things I didn't care about have come into play," he told me sadly. "In hindsight, I wished I'd listened. I developed a cataract in my right eye due to Prednisone. My bones have always been low density and there's a pretty significant risk of osteoporosis." He has not been in a relationship and, at 23, lived with his parents until he could get back on his feet.

Gina, 26 when we spoke, enumerated her side effects with a certain detachment and wry humor. "You can get really manic, you can get super depressed, acne all over your face and body, swelling in your joints and limbs. I get ADD, joint pain, insatiable hunger and your brain chemistry goes off. It's crazy. I get heart palpitations. Can't catch your breath. Can't sleep. You're not tired, which actually helps around finals. Can't absorb calcium, so you lose muscle. It's fun to tell people you're on steroids and watch their expressions."

Remicade is another powerful and often extremely effective medication, but it carries a very slight chance of causing lymphoma later in life. Statistically, the chances of this occurring are extremely small, but the very mention of the risk causes terror in parents who fear they unintentionally might be creating larger problems for their child in the long term in an effort to control symptoms in the present.

Remicade doesn't work for everyone, but when it does, it can turn your life around vastly for the better. But it is expensive, thousands of dollars per infusion, a cost that is sometimes subsidized by the drug company or the hospital. Some patients with whom I spoke said Remicade and Humira were end-of-the-line medications for them. If they didn't work, surgery was the only option. So the stakes are high.

Karen struggled to get her teenaged son, Joseph, to accept that he had Crohn's disease for life and to assume responsibility for taking his medicine. Her use of the pronoun "we" implies how strongly parents identify with their children's illness and how tough are the decisions about medications. "We did the 6MP first, then the Pentasa and that wasn't quieting anything down," she said. "So we decided Remicade was the best way." Remicade was a hard choice, because Karen's father suffered from non-Hodgkin's lymphoma and Karen feared that Joseph was particularly vulnerable to this side effect because of the family history. However, as a surgical technician, she tried to see the situation through the eyes of a health care worker. She decided that the risks were worth the benefits, because she understood that the pharmaceutical company has to "disclose every possible thing." Karen sat Joseph down and gave him the choice of how to take it. "'Eventually, you're going to have to take care of yourself as an adult," she told him. Joseph decided to get an infusion of Remicade in a hospital every eight weeks instead of injecting himself at home every two weeks. It has worked so well that he feels the disease has disappeared. "Now that I'm on Remicade," Joseph told me, "I feel like I don't have Crohn's anymore."

Enemas and the Art of Submission

Those of us who have endured over-the-counter enemas as short term fixes for constipation have to replay the unpleasantness with medicinal enemas for ulcerative colitis. Medicinal enemas deliver cortisone locally to the rectum and lower colon to heal the inflamed area without introducing the potent drug into the bloodstream.

Just as with over-the-counter enemas, however, the problem is that you need to hold the liquid inside the lower colon as long as possible to give the enema a chance to work. Because the colon is inflamed, it is extremely difficult not to give in to the cramps that want to expel the liquid too quickly. Melissa, 28, realized that if she didn't hold the liquid long enough for the medicine to do its work, it literally meant $18 down the toilet.

Enemas interfere with social life in awkward ways. The time it takes to hold in the enema is time you're taking away from being with your friends or your date. Joel recalled trying to balance a relationship with his then-girlfriend with taking the enema. "We were hanging out in the living room. I wanted to ravish her. Instead, I'm saying, 'How about you stay in the living room and I go into the bedroom and do my thing, and I'll see you in a half hour? I need to be in this quiet space.' It's very tricky," he said sadly. "It instantly ages you."

Rachel, who underwent an ileostomy, a surgical opening in the intestinal wall, because of Crohn's, still took cortisone enemas to suppress inflammation near her rectum. "Everybody likes to be in control of everything in our lives," she said. "Every night for the past four years I've taken enemas and, some nights, I put them in and they won't stay in. They squirt foam up your body. It's horrible."

On the other hand, the local cortisone can sometimes help patients stay off oral steroids. Diane, who was diagnosed in high school, takes a steroid enema for her ulcerative colitis. She observed, "It's amazing how some things that were so gross to you at some point become routine. Enemas used to horrify me. Now I don't care. I'll do anything not to take steroids."

Medications that Stop Working

Some medications for IBD work like miracle drugs, then suddenly may not work at all. The stories I heard about the search for the medication that will take away symptoms forever constituted nothing less than sagas. When a medication works, it brings hope and optimism for the future. When the same medication stops working, patients feel disappointed and pessimistic. The cycle is crazy making. Patients become cynical about the possibility of ever suppressing their symptoms as they cycle through drug after drug.

Remicade is particularly frustrating, because after it has worked so well, some patients became allergic to the mouse protein in it and they have to stop. One such patient was Rachel, who cycled through several drugs without a positive effect until she went on Remicade. "They just couldn't get it under control," she said of her Crohn's disease, which made her temporarily drop out of university in England. "They tried every drug under the sun. I injected myself and they hooked me up to things. Either the drugs did not work at all, or gave me false hope by working for six months. Remicade worked on and off for three years. Most of the time it worked really well. But then I got severe side effects on my skin: ulcers, really bad infections and uveitis, an eye inflammation, that destroyed some vision in one eye."

Kelly was another who thought Remicade was a permanent answer to her colitis. As a college freshman, she decided not to take the steroid suppositories and she became sicker and sicker by taking no medication at all. She was prescribed the anti-inflammatories Entocort and Asacol, but nothing worked until Remicade. At first, it acted like a miracle drug. The symptoms stopped for almost

18 months. Then she went into anaphylactic shock after she developed an allergy to Remicade's mouse protein. To make things more confusing, Kelly then went through cycles of being symptom free on no medication before her disease flared again. When we spoke, Kelly, 25, was taking Methotrexate, a powerful drug used for cancer patients as well as for IBD. It wiped out her symptoms and her immune system and exhausted her. Each day, when she leaves her teaching job, she goes directly home to sleep.

Medication and Vacations

Taking medication is not a social enterprise. Unless you are young and your parents are part of the process, you take your enemas and pills apart from your friends and family. Taking enemas becomes tricky when you go on vacation, because you're usually sharing a room with a friend or a partner. It is also important to calculate the number of pills you will need. If side effects from medication should occur, you are isolated from your friends at the very time you want to be playing.

Once, I traveled to Puerto Rico and lay on the beach, soaking up the warm sun with abandon. I'd forgotten that exposing myself to too much sun would activate a side effect of Azulfadine, the sulfa drug I took three times daily to keep my colitis under control. So when my friends left for dinner, I stayed in bed, possessed by uncontrollable shaking from chills that lasted for several hours.

Joel was vacationing in Cancun, Mexico with two friends when he realized he had miscounted the number of pills he'd brought with him. "When you leave the house, you have to add to your life's tasks to count your pills," he said. Joel was afraid he'd develop diarrhea and he decided he needed to get more pills. He left the tourist area and entered a seedy neighborhood where he found a pharmacy. He spied a book on the counter cataloguing a list of medications and found his prescription as an over-the-counter drug. "It saved my vacation," Joel remembered with gratitude. "It was awesome."

Compromising the Immune System

Because IBD causes inflammation, many of the drugs used to combat it are designed to suppress your body's immune system so your digestive system doesn't overreact to perceived assailants such as food and healthy bacteria, thus creating more inflammation. The disadvantage is that because your immunity is suppressed, it is not as available to fight off bacterial infections and viruses. The drugs create a vicious cycle. Many patients become more susceptible to flare-ups from IBD after they catch a virus or a bacterial infection because their gut doesn't know when to stop fighting.

Scott got a virus every semester of college. "I'd been on Methotrexate, Remicade, and Prednisone since 2004," he told me. Because his immunity is so compromised, he worried, exaggerating for effect, that "getting a virus is a death sentence." On medical leave from graduate school, where he studied environmental policy, Scott wasn't sure if he would return, not because he couldn't handle the work, but because he feared catching a virus from the other students.

"It puts me in a position where I'm always at risk of flaring," he said. "A sneezing, coughing virus will trigger my symptoms. When I get any type of flu, it triggers my immune system to become overactive. Once a virus kicks the immune system on for people with IBD, it doesn't register that it needs to turn off."

CONCLUSION

Many patients with IBD remain stabilized on one medication or a cocktail of drugs for many years with minimal side effects. However, many patients I interviewed had more complicated interactions with their medications.

After reading about others who experience difficulties, those of you who have encountered success with medication may feel grateful for your good fortune. In listening to story after story, I certainly felt thankful that I was able to remain on Azulfadine for 30 years with minimal side effects. I maintained the maximum dose through good times and bad, because most of the time, I realized that even when I felt good, the disease was dormant and by no means gone. I credited my remission in small part to all the emotional and psychological work I had done, but mostly to Azulfadine's ability to keep my symptoms in check.

However, those of you who contend with the mercurial and distressing effects of medication may take consolation in knowing that many others confront the same problems. It is scant comfort, of course, when you are suffering with both IBD and its treatments, but any reassurance that you are not an outlier goes a long way toward helping you to accept your situation, even if you do so ruefully.

CHAPTER SIX

Navigating Elementary School Through College

I always tried to keep my healthy persona separate from my sick persona. I lost a lot of friends in middle school and high school, who had no idea that any of this was going on. I felt isolated for a long time.

— **Jamie Weinstein**

Secrets are toxic. Secrets cause the brain to engage in a fight with itself, according to David Eagleman, a neuroscientist at the Baylor College of Medicine, who found that one part of the brain wants to tell the secret and the other wants to keep it hidden. (Eagleman, 2009) Yet many young people with IBD live alone with the secret of their disease. And the place where they live with it the most, day in and day out, is school.

Aside from schoolwork, the major undertaking from kindergarten through college is to develop emotionally as a human being. Every young person's identity is fluid. Approval from classmates means everything. Internally, small humiliations can balloon into major catastrophes. Friendships and social groups shift and those fluctuations can prompt insecurity or self-doubt, even when health is good.

But IBD can create a wall, setting one apart from healthy friends. The issues encountered by students are surprisingly the same whether they are in kindergarten or college. Students who try to keep IBD secret from their classmates soldier on alone through pain, cramping, and urgency, without support, and without anyone commiserating with them.

Young children in particular feel overwhelmed by a diagnosis they don't entirely understand. Very young children don't even know how to answer when asked what is wrong with them, and they can barely pronounce the full name of the disease that is stealing their childhood.

Shawn, 27 when we spoke, has lived with Crohn's disease since he was 5. He offered his perspective about why he kept it a secret in school. "I did not want to be treated any differently," he told me. "I wanted to be just like any other kid at school, which must have been the reason I never said anything to my friends. Part of it was I didn't understand the disease myself. I just knew that when I ate food, I felt stomach pain and needed to go to the bathroom. It's embarrassing to say I have to go to the bathroom several times a day with stomach pain. It's not something a child wants to share with his friends."

Shawn could say all this when he was 27. It is almost impossible for young people to articulate the reasons why they don't want classmates to know they have IBD. But here are a few of the many concerns I gleaned from talking with parents and young people with IBD:

They wonder whether they will be bullied or, at the very least, teased. They worry whether they will be able to leave the classroom quickly enough to make it to the bathroom or whether they will have an embarrassing accident that leaves them exposed and humiliated. They struggle to figure out how to communicate that IBD involves much more than an upset stomach, but they don't want to offer embarrassing details. They want to fit in with their healthy friends, who eat pizza and drink soda or beer whenever they want. They wish they could be part of their school's physical and social activities and not be limited by their illness. In every respect, they don't want to stand out.

Even if a young child is open about IBD, it is an invisible disease. Other than the effects of Prednisone, IBD is usually not evident to others.

Trinity was diagnosed with ulcerative colitis at 8 after five years of mysterious symptoms, as described in Chapter One. Her mother obtained a 504 plan, which refers to Section 504 of the Americans with Disabilities Act. It states that no one with a physical or mental impairment that substantially limits major life activities can be excluded from participating in school. A 504 plan, however effective it may be in securing a place in the classroom, cannot protect a student with IBD from being harassed by fellow students. After taking Prednisone, Trinity's face took on a moon shape and she suddenly gained weight. A group of girls wrote "fat" and "cow" on her desk and rewrote it as soon as Trinity erased it. The girls thought Trinity was pretending to be sick, and they couldn't understand the school's accommodations for her, since other than the weight gain, she had no outward signs of disease.

Some students with IBD have to deal with the torments of classmates. But they also have to deal with school rules that work against them. Many schools have strict guidelines that prevent students from leaving in the middle of class to use a bathroom, particularly during tests. Even during an everyday class, teachers may become annoyed and inflexible when a student with IBD raises his or her hand multiple times asking to go to the bathroom.

When Stephanie was in elementary school, she couldn't explain to her classmates what was wrong with her. Diagnosed with ulcerative colitis at 10, she couldn't even pronounce the name of her disease after being hospitalized with it for two weeks. In high school, her teacher and principal were both unenlightened and stubborn. She was taking a test and she raised her hand to ask to go to the bathroom. Her teacher refused to let her leave. "She's probably thinking, 'She's got her period,' Stephanie said, "but I had a flare-up." She lost control. "It was everywhere. It was a mess." Someone gave her a sweater to cover herself as she walked out of the classroom feeling humiliated. She heard her classmates whispering, 'What's wrong with her? Why did it smell when she walked past us?' After the incident, Stephanie's mother visited the school principal and her daughter's teachers and gave them pamphlets about ulcerative colitis from the Crohn's and Colitis Foundation of America (CCFA). In front of her mother, the principal, a nun, threw the packet into the wastebasket.

Carolyn suffered the humiliation that kids with IBD fear. Diagnosed at 14, she lost so much weight so quickly from Crohn's while in sixth grade that she described being "horribly bullied" for it. She was 5'1" and 68 pounds. "Everybody thought I was anorexic," she said. "People would shout at me. I would end up eating in the bathroom if I ate at all. People I didn't even know dropped food on my head. I tried to tell them I was hurting and wasn't trying to make myself sick. I was so thin it looked like I was about to fall. I tried to talk to the administration and they did nothing." Her mother took her out of that pernicious environment and transferred her to a private school, where the bullying stopped.

Kathy pulled her son Paul out of his elementary school "because they wouldn't work with his limitations. I was so disappointed," she said. "I didn't get a 504 plan when he was diagnosed. I felt it was a Christian school and they'd work with him. The teachers were accommodating in letting him go to the bathroom when he needed to go. The lunch aides wouldn't. My son isn't a rule breaker, so when the aides said no one could go to the bathroom, I talked to the aides and the principal, and they said he could be an exception to the rule. But Paul felt sure that he would still get in trouble and he'd stand out."

Robert's mother, Linda, was still angry and aggrieved when she recalled how the teachers in her son's Long Island, N.Y. high school were unsympathetic to her son's condition. When Robert was hospitalized with Crohn's in tenth grade and had to miss six weeks of school, one of the teachers confronted his mother when she came to the school to pick up some books. "I heard he was out partying," the teacher said to his mother. "I lost it," Linda said. "Maybe if the teacher hadn't said 'partying' I'd have been okay. Maybe if he weren't so sick, I wouldn't have been so mad."

Missing School

The contrast between the life one leads before IBD and the life one leads after it is almost too stark to digest. It is not uncommon for students with severe IBD to spend weeks or months away from the classroom when they become too sick to be in school. It's medically necessary, of course, but their absence disrupts social connections, extracurricular sports, and other activities and makes people with IBD even more insecure than they were before.

When Clinton was in seventh grade in British Columbia, Canada, he worried that his sickness was taking a toll on his friendships. "It's a time you're trying to figure everything out," he said. "I was out of school for tests and hospitalized several times. I was away from my friends, and they didn't understand what was going on with me." Clinton was afraid to go on field trips because he would urgently need a bathroom and he didn't want to have an accident. But he went. On one field trip, he sat on a bench and started to bawl. "I was so fed up with it. I just wanted to be normal. No special disease, just a normal kid who would blend in with everybody else. I didn't want to stand out."

Of the many people whom I interviewed, few have grappled with as many emotional problems associated with their IBD as Edward. Short in stature, articulate, and beset with depression, Edward struggled to make his way in the world as a young adult.

Edward has a serious case of Crohn's disease that was diagnosed when he was 14. He was so sick, he had to withdraw from eighth grade. Classmates at his small private middle school did not disappoint him — they dedicated their graduation to him. Life wasn't so bad. He was tutored at home, so he could rise late, do some work, and then watch movies and baseball on television.

Those halcyon days ended when he entered a large, competitive public high school. Before walking in the door for the first time, he anticipated that his classmates would stay away from him, because, thanks to Prednisone, he looked puffy. But that didn't happen right away. "People were actually nice freshman year. I was funny. Nobody makes fun of a funny fat kid," he said wryly. "A lot of people knew me. I felt good. I felt like I was part of something. I was writing for the school newspaper. I was really sick, but in terms of my emotional state, things were great."

When Edward had to miss months of school because he was too ill, however, he felt forgotten and alienated. Back at school after the hiatus, he would nod to someone he knew but they wouldn't recognize or acknowledge him, partly because he had stopped taking Prednisone and lost weight.

He became stressed and depressed, and that exacerbated his IBD symptoms, he said. His Crohn's became too serious for him to stay in school. He was homebound and isolated once more. He tried going back one more time. He lasted for a single class. "It was one of the worst days of school I ever had," he said. "I hated it. I absolutely hated being back there." Edward never went back. He preferred being tutored at home to confronting cold shoulders at school.

Facing college

College can be a time of exploration and independence, of making new friends, of experimenting with freedom from parents and studying new subjects more deeply than ever before. Except for people with IBD.

With IBD, college is a time of dealing with your illness largely on your own, without parents nearby. While some roommates are considerate and sensitive, others seemed to sniff out a problem and pounce on it. Indeed, sometimes the social failures that occurred in high school carry over to college.

Laura was 18 and two weeks into the second semester of her freshman year at Pennsylvania State University when she suddenly developed symptoms that turned out to be ulcerative colitis. She went back to school for two more years, but she was so sick, she withdrew to go home and lie on the couch. She asked the question posed by many people afflicted with disease: "Why me?"

Laura wondered which friends would stick by her and which would forget her. "I went back to visit," she said. "I had a moon face and acne" from the Prednisone. She was ashamed. She didn't feel normal. She felt always on the outside because of her illness. Her mother, Kim, kept a diary during that period. She wrote that it bothered Laura that some of her friends didn't seem to care. Kim understood it differently. "One of your college friends called for you one day, but you weren't home. He told me that he hadn't talked to you in a while. He told me that it wasn't that he didn't care, he just didn't know what to say to you and how to handle it. The other thing that ticked you off was when people would say it was all in your head. They said you must be under a lot of stress. How uneducated people were!"

It is intuitive that college students will react more maturely than those in elementary school and high school, particularly toward anyone whose appearance is different or who has odd bathroom habits. So when meanness toward people with IBD occurs in college, it's almost shocking. But even some college students tormented people with IBD in ways that sadly echoed elementary school bullying.

It was traumatic for Chava to be intermittently incontinent in college. "It's bad enough when you're young, but for someone at 19, 20, 21, it was devastating," she said. "I couldn't go out. Even going to class became challenging at times. I couldn't talk about it to anybody." During her senior year, she had a "horrible experience with a girl I shared a bathroom with. Every time I went to the bathroom, she was on the other side of the door yelling and swearing at me. She'd yell, 'I can't believe I have to listen to these noises!'"

Kelly was diagnosed as a freshman at Ohio State University. During her last three years of college, she lived with roommates who were unreliable and unsympathetic when she became medically vulnerable. "It was a big thing for them to drop me off at the hospital," she said. "I don't know why they wouldn't do those kind of things. They all had cars." When she left a class twice to go to the bathroom, a roommate asked, "Why? Didn't you go before?" adding, "It's embarrassing, you get up to go so much." "Girls are mean," Kelly said tightly. "They would talk about me behind my back." Inexplicably, Kelly lived with these roommates throughout college. She doesn't know why she stayed with them. "It was almost like I was sucked into their game. It was ridiculous now that I look back on it."

Psychologist Kodman-Jones believes that a snappy comeback in response to the teaser or bully can make them go away. "It's how you handle the bullying," she said. "If you have a good comeback, after a while they stop because you're not going to take it. There are teens who'll say, 'Oh, that's so gross.' You answer, 'Yes, that's gross. Get a life. Everybody poops. Everybody farts. They stink. It's what happens. Get over it.' You have to be a little tougher. I work a lot with kids who've been teased about something. You have to work with it. It's a reality. We all get teased."

Some college students with IBD find that the stress both socially and academically is too much to handle. They choose either to transfer to a school closer to home or to live at home and commute so that they'll have access to a private toilet, and so they'll feel less self-conscious about making loud noises or emitting smelly odors.

Amanda had moderate Crohn's disease while in high school, but it erupted into major flare-ups when she entered a college two hours away from home. "Being there wasn't great for my stomach," she recalled. "I went there for one semester. They had two stalls for ten girls and you had to use your ID badge to go to the bathroom. So when you had to run, it was not that great. That's why I chose to transfer to a school closer to home and lived at home."

Relieving Emotional Distress

Despite such distressing memories, the overwhelming message I took away from speaking with young people with IBD is that when they took the risk and disclosed what was really going on, the vast majority found support and sympathy, both from classmates and school staff. And, equally as affirming, they got the equivalent of a big yawn, a nonchalant acceptance that showed them that their disease was no big deal and didn't affect their friendships. The anxiety that had been festering inside them bore no relationship to reality.

For example, it took two years before Nicole, diagnosed at 9, told anyone she had Crohn's disease. Then she moved to a new town in New Jersey, made different friends, and decided the time was right to open up. She called a friend and told her she had Crohn's. Her friend said, "Okay." It was a non-issue. Nicole was relieved that she wasn't going to lose friends over it, although she still carried residual embarrassment. "Colitis is not the most pleasant disease to explain to people even now," she said, a college student when we spoke. "I sometimes feel people are a little grossed out, as they probably should be. I have no idea how people will react. I would rather tell them I am sick and have them think I had the flu than say, 'I have stomachaches. I have to go the bathroom 100 times a day.'"

She now talks about IBD in a way that tells enough but not too much. She will answer people who ask her about Crohn's disease this way: "Most people have good cells and bad cells, and to keep you healthy, the good cells attack the bad cells. But when you have an autoimmune disease, the good cells attack all the cells, and that's what's going on in my large intestine."

"Usually at that point," she said, "that's enough for them."

As Nicole indicated, students can liberate themselves from their misery once they start talking openly about their IBD.

After years of feeling humiliated at the mention of his illness, Joseph experimented with being more open about his Crohn's disease at the end of his sophomore year of high school. He started talking about his recent surgery. He told everybody that he has Crohn's and that parts of his intestines are diseased and that his stomach bothers him and he has diarrhea. His classmates' response? "They're just like, 'That stinks' or, 'Oh, really? One of my family members has it.' A lot more people have it than I thought."

Scott, diagnosed at 12, managed to avoid discussing his ulcerative colitis with friends because he was fearful of seeming like a freak. He was alone with it until, inadvertently, at the end of his freshman year at American University, the game was up. Someone opened the drawer in his bedside table and saw that it was filled with medications. "I was caught," he said. "My secret was revealed." Out of necessity or loneliness, Scott made the leap to openness. He hoped that if he became more forthcoming about his Crohn's, he could make closer connections. He developed friendships with classmates who did not have colitis, but who were interested enough to openly discuss it with him. "That was nice," he said. "I really didn't want a group of friends who could not handle the information."

When students incorporate IBD as part of their identity, without internally letting it take over their lives, it is a boost to their self-image and their ego. Perhaps not coincidentally, their classmates and teachers often respond with compassion and understanding.

In Josh's home, perhaps because IBD was something the family had always lived with, everyone had a strong attitude that it was okay to talk about farting, pooping, and letting it rip. This openness at home transferred to Josh's life at school and helped him to lose any shred of embarrassment he may have had. He was frank about his Crohn's disease, and his honesty, in turn, created an atmosphere in which he could find support at school. In his high school, he used a code word that meant he couldn't get up without losing control of his bowels and that communicated to his buddies, "Pick me up and get me out of here."

Jacque, Josh's mother, attributed the receptivity of Josh's classmates and others at school to her blunt approach with them. "I reached out to the high school nurse and printed out the information pamphlet from the CCFA," she told me. "I introduced myself at the open house, and said, 'If he's ever told he can't go to the bathroom, hell hath no fury like the fury they'll see in me.'" Problem solved. This is not to minimize the obstacles that parents have to confront with teachers and administrators. But the message is this: Sometimes, bluntness and covert threats work.

So does unabashed openness. Shawna had a 504 plan that smoothed her way through elementary school. She was diagnosed with IBD at age 6 and had no trouble accepting the disease because she could barely remember her life without it. "I told everyone," she said. "It was like, 'I got a puppy. I got a disease.' My therapist helped me figure out how to tell people the nice way rather than give them the gutsy details. In sixth grade, I started a dance-athon to raise money for IBD. One kid came because his mother had it. The more people I tell, the more people I meet who have it or know someone else who does."

Tiffany was diagnosed at 16. She feels "very fortunate to have been in a private school. They were extremely understanding," she told me. "They went out of their way to make sure I could continue to be in school. I could come and go as I wanted. All my teachers gave me extra tutoring if I needed it, because I'd constantly miss class or fall asleep in class. We were constantly trying to wean me off Prednisone, which was not successful. My parents wrote a letter saying if I start crying spontaneously or falling asleep, don't say anything."

Maggie, who underwent ostomy surgery as a junior in high school for Crohn's, found understanding and outreach from her public high school while she was out of school for two months. Her teachers went to her house and taught her after school. "I hear about all these people having problems with school and needing help," she said, but in her case, she added, "Everybody was very understanding."

Trinity, whose problems with classmates are detailed above, found that her school responded positively after her colon was surgically removed and she received a J-pouch. The principal visited her in the hospital. Classmates sent get well cards. Still, Trinity was worried that she would be forgotten because of all the time away from school. Her fears were unfounded. "For a public school, they did fabulously," her mother, LeAnne, said, adding that Trinity was able to use the bathroom as often as she needed. When we spoke, Trinity had the same concerns as any student in fourth grade. "When I got back to school, I got the student of the month award. I was pretty happy about that. They call your name and everyone claps for you and you get a small pencil that says, 'Student of the Month.' Although, I'm getting a little annoyed, because every year, I've gotten student of the month. I'd like to get a music award."

Marjorie, who was from Boston, knew no one with IBD when she was in high school, but that changed when she went to Carleton College in Minnesota. "I said I had Crohn's and I got assigned to a double with a bathroom," she said. One night in the fall of her freshman year, someone mentioned he had Crohn's, and someone else said she had Crohn's and Maggie felt empowered to say she had Crohn's. "College was great, because I got to have this conversation," she said. "I'd never had a conversation [about Crohn's] with anyone else before."

Krystal, who developed symptoms of virulent Crohn's in third grade, developed a way of thinking about it that guides her to this day — an insight that ties together all of these positive and negative experiences. She recognized that the best offense against teasing and mistreatment was to concede that IBD is a fact of one's life and to come to terms with it. "I think the most important thing is to accept your situation and be okay with having Crohn's and having an ostomy," said Krystal, who has both. "People can't ridicule you for something you're okay with. They can't make fun of something that you accept. It just doesn't work."

How to Advocate for Yourself

Without a doubt, self-acceptance is easier said than done. However, one way to begin accepting yourself is to act as if you do, even when you are feeling insecure. In short, to quote a cliché that's a cliché because it's true, fake it until you make it.

The Crohn's and Colitis Foundation has offered some practical ways to inform teachers and administrators about your IBD:

1. Have your doctor write a note to the school staff notifying them of your IBD. Make sure the note includes information about your need to use the bathroom often, if that's the case, or about any other symptoms that may interfere with class work.

2. If you are a student, talk to your teacher privately. This can be the first step in your emergence from behind the mask of making believe you're like everyone else. The vast majority of teachers will be understanding and empathetic. It's a good way to practice talking to someone who may never have heard of Crohn's disease or ulcerative colitis or who doesn't understand how all-consuming these conditions can be. If you are reluctant, ask a parent or guardian to accompany you and get the conversation going. Then, speak up for yourself.

3. Ask your teacher(s) to allow you to leave class to use the bathroom without having to raise your hand to ask permission. Perhaps you can agree on a hand signal to notify the teacher of your need to leave immediately. Perhaps the teacher will agree to let you simply get up and go without any notification. To establish trust, do not abuse the privilege. Go only when you have to go. If you encounter any resistance along the way and your condition is serious, consider obtaining a 504 plan (see explanation above.)

CHAPTER SEVEN
Nontraditional Treatments for IBD

I am most certainly a junk food addict and look at where it has gotten me: I am unable to move from the toilet for more than an hour before nature — hideous, hideous nature — beckons me.

— *A Recluse's Guide*
by Ben Brandfon (unpublished novel)

It would be wonderful if your predilection for junk foods or other unhealthy eating could be held directly responsible for your IBD. If only IBD were as uncomplicated as that. It also would be ideal if alternative measures, such as acupuncture, yoga, and herbs consistently relieved the symptoms of IBD. Alas, IBD confounds the many patients and parents who try to find surefire approaches to treatments.

Driven by stories of unconventional measures that work, patients and parents find ample reasons to hope for discovering a miracle on the Internet or through word of mouth. They encounter stories about restrictive diets, herbal remedies, and feats of healing when hope was all but lost. And, so, with or without consulting their physician, they enter the complicated world of alternative strategies to impose control on the obstinate symptoms of IBD.

So seductive are patients' stories about how radical dietary changes or alternative approaches cured or substantially downgraded the symptoms of their Crohn's or colitis that I found myself wanting to share them with readers. However, much more to the point of the psychological and social impact of IBD is to explore how patients and their families are affected emotionally and socially by their quest outside the realm of their doctor's prescriptions, and by their failure or success to find the relief they are seeking.

Complementary and Alternative Medicine

First, let's define the terms. Complementary and alternative medicine (CAM) encompass therapies beyond the bounds of conventional medicine, boundaries that are becoming more fluid as doctors begin to see the value — or, at least, the absence of harm — in many of the measures their patients have been using for years.

According to several studies conducted in North America and Europe, about half of IBD patients turn to alternative therapies and nutritional supplements such as probiotics, fish oil, herbal medications, marijuana, (Lal, Simon, 2011) yoga, acupuncture, and homeopathy. Among their reasons were ineffective medicines, inadequate feelings of control over IBD and the deleterious side effects from conventional drug treatment. Most patients consult their physicians before engaging in these therapies, but some abandon conventional medicines altogether, using alternative measures alone with mixed results.

The primary impetus that drives patients to explore CAM is to restore a feeling of control, a feeling that is often lost in the maelstrom of medicines, side effects and worsening symptoms. Restricting what goes into your mouth represents an attempt to contain a disease that may otherwise feel unmanageable. And perceiving that you are more in charge of your own treatment is empowering. The sheer will and dogged pursuit of a diet or alternative measures that may take away abhorrent symptoms is heroic when it works and poignant when it doesn't.

"When you feel out of control with your disease, you try to control your environment," said psychologist Kodman-Jones, who has 20 years of experience working with young people with IBD. "You say, 'I can't control anything. I'm going to break all the rules.' You can be bitter. Or you can do everything you know to do and say, 'I'm doing the best I can.'"

Diets

Eating is one of life's great pleasures. Being deprived of doing it with thoughtless abandon is an emotional stressor on people with IBD. No matter what you believe about the interaction of the foods you eat and your disease, you will never again eat in a carefree way without even a thought to the price you might pay.

In retrospect, I regret my impetuous attitude toward food when I had ulcerative colitis. I responded to my helplessness by breaking all the rules. I ate anything I wanted, and I suffered for it. It is almost a cliché to talk about patients who deny they have IBD. But when I went out with friends, I pretended I was normal and paid later with stomach cramps and bloody diarrhea. Then, one day, I had to stop eating pizza and drinking beer. My flare-ups had become so serious that my doctor took me off all regular food and put me on a liquid protein drink, gradually advancing me to jarred baby food. It took a considerable amount of time to arrest the flare-ups. I would like to say I learned my lesson, but the truth is that I never disciplined my eating in deference to colitis.

Given my history, I listened with particular interest to other patients describe their struggles with food and symptoms.

Despite the CCFA's unconditional assertions to the contrary, many patients suspect that eating carelessly caused their disease. Ben, who has Crohn's disease, put it this way, "Did I do this to myself somehow because I ate badly? I never had the greatest diet or eating habits. Maybe, if I had taken better care of myself..."

Convinced that their diet influences their IBD, other patients try to manage an internal battle between food cravings and their determination to combat their disease. Alisa had a hard time staying on a restricted diet, because of the way it interfered with her social life as well as the sheer difficulty of adhering to it. She went on a restricted diet because she had heard about people who had cured their IBD with diet. Alisa's doctor dismissed the role of diet and told her to expect to be on pills forever.

But Alisa chose to go on a restricted diet anyway. Like many people with IBD, her adherence to the diet wavers, because she is married, she has a social life, and she is prone to food cravings. She careens between eating everything and then eating nothing in order to perform a "cleanse," a modified liquid fast of juice, tea, and lemonade made with maple syrup and cayenne pepper. Proponents claim that a cleanse can detoxify the body. There is no scientific evidence of that, or that it achieves anything beyond a temporary weight loss.

After a cleanse, Alisa would eat only plant-based foods. After a time, she would grow weary of all the food restrictions she had put herself on. She would throw them off and ingest everything she wanted, including alcohol, which triggered her colitis symptoms. She seesawed between remission and flare-ups. One time, she said, she had a "pretty bad flare and a hemorrhoid. It was not a pretty picture, but I had so much fun, I'd do it again."

The patience, discipline, and determination that it takes to follow a strict dietary regimen is obviously not for everyone, no matter how much a patient wants to get well. Following such diets becomes even more onerous when there is no guarantee of any positive effect on their disease. When patients dutifully follow a diet and see no improvement, they can feel resentful and hopeless.

"I wish I had the tenacity to endure one of those all-natural diets that supposedly cure Crohn's," said Jason. "And, yes, I did give it a try. I threw out all my bread and bought nut flour. I had to make everything from scratch, which wasn't easy for someone whose idea of cooking started and ended with the microwave. I stayed up all night making that special probiotic yogurt, checking on it every hour to make sure the temperature was just right. This was supposed to be the best thing for you," he said. Then he added, suddenly addressing his Crohn's, "And how did you react? You pitched a fit."

However, Shira is a true believer in the power of diet, combined with yoga and acupuncture, to positively affect her ulcerative colitis. She was scared into taking control of her disease when she discovered her grandmother had had colon cancer and her mother's personal trainer warned her that she would one day develop cancer if she didn't take steps to alleviate her disease. "From that day forward, I made a change," she told me. "I'm gluten free. I do eat meat, but always grass-fed, organic [meat], and I don't eat a lot of it. I eat dairy very rarely. I do acupuncture twice a month, I'm a yoga teacher and I meditate. In 2009, I had a colonoscopy. The doctor told me the colitis was 11 centimeters in my colon. In 2011, it was at 3 centimeters. Basically I know that everybody says there's no cure, yada yada. I feel like I'm on that road."

Doctors and CAM

Doctors often refer their patients to nutritionists for advice about what they should eat. But the general attitude of doctors regarding diet is vague at best. Their standard advice to patients is to refrain from eating what makes them feel sick and to eat everything else. They note, if questioned, that there is no scientific data proving that diet contributes to flare-ups.

This, for example, is the position of Dr. Steven Werlin, who practices gastroenterology at the Children's Hospital of Wisconsin in Milwaukee. "It's okay if it doesn't make you sick," he said. "We have dieticians who are available to work with our patients. But I don't believe in a lot of restrictions."

Werlin's attitude is supported by the CCFA. "Patients often believe that their disease is caused by, and can be cured by diet. Unfortunately, that seems to be too simplistic an approach, which is not supported by clinical and scientific data. Diet can certainly affect symptoms of these diseases, and may play some role in the underlying inflammatory process, but it appears not to be the major factor in the inflammatory process."

The issue that plagues many people trying to determine what to eat is, if diet can "certainly affect symptoms of these diseases," as the CCFA says, why won't physicians help patients figure out what to eat?

Addressing the uncertainty over the effect of diet on IBD would enhance an atmosphere of honesty in the relationship between doctors and patients. Doctors could acknowledge that they themselves have little knowledge of nutrition (only 30 percent of medical schools require even one nutrition course); and they could inform their patients about how little is known in general about the effect of diet on IBD, rather than claim, as many doctors do, that diet is irrelevant.

When patients become sicker despite medications and doctors tell them they can eat anything that agrees with them, many patients lose faith in medicine and turn to potentially harmful restrictive diets. One gastroenterologist, addressing her colleagues, adopts a tone at once pleading and slightly scolding as she appeals to them to pay more attention to the effect of diet on IBD for the sake of the doctor-patient relationship.

"The question that IBD patients ask most often and want to spend the most time discussing is, "Doctor, what should I eat?" wrote Dr. Sunanda Kane, professor of medicine in the Division of Gastroenterology at the Mayo Clinic in Rochester, Minnesota. "During office visits, the feeling is that no attention is paid to eating. When the physician says, 'It doesn't matter what you eat,' it leads to patient dissatisfaction and distrust.

"Since patients can tell when certain foods are bothersome, they then distrust their healthcare provider and perhaps their recommendations for other disease-management issues," Dr. Kane continued. "In addition, patients then often turn to experimentation with fad or restriction diets. Patients who are not counseled and believe that certain foods cause disease or lead to aggravated symptoms may avoid foods that actually are beneficial, causing worse health due to vitamin deficiencies and malnutrition. The scientific literature is conflicting in terms of the role of food, which does not help," she concluded. (Kane, 2014)

Another factor in the distance between patients and doctors is the reluctance of patients to share with their physicians the details of their ventures into unconventional treatments. An in-depth questionnaire given to 16 doctors and nurses by the Karolinska Institute in Sweden in 2013 about their attitudes toward CAM found the following: "The participants perceived that patients were reluctant to talk about CAM and did not spontaneously inform them that they used such methods." One of the medical researchers surmised that his patients were afraid that this information would be treated with contempt. "I think they don't want to make [fools] of themselves in front of the doctor by relating that they use CAM," he said. (Lindberg, 2013)

Parents who haven't lost faith in traditional medicine try to find a balance between that and self-management through diet. Kim is one of these. She lives in Western Pennsylvania at the New Life Bible Camp, which is run by her husband. Her daughter Chloe's colitis hadn't subsided in the two years after her diagnosis at age 6. Concern for her daughter led Kim to take things into her own hands.

"We understand diet is not supposed to cure ulcerative colitis, but it's not even included in our treatment at all," she said with frustration in her voice. She tried in vain to find a medical professional "who is not totally swayed in one direction or the other, someone who's able to include a diet that's healthy and shows promise. People are on one side, where all they want is a diet, and the other side, where all they want is to throw pills at you. Nobody's looking at the whole body instead of a set of symptoms."

Kim abandoned going to a physician at the Children's Hospital of Pittsburgh because when she asked about the best nutrition for colitis, all he could recommend was a liquid protein shake. "Sorry, I don't want her to drink Boost," Kim said dryly, referring to a brand of shake. "There are diets that some people say work and I don't know why they don't suggest that in conjunction with medications," she said. "On the flip side, I've read that some alternative therapies sound like hocus-pocus." Back and forth, she volleyed with herself, reflecting the ambivalence many families feel.

While some IBD nutrition books sounded promising to Kim, she found others to be antagonistic to the medical community, claiming that they were trying to gouge people's pocketbooks. "I don't agree with that either," Kim said. "They're all standing at opposite sides, throwing stones at each other." All this conflicting information leaves patients and their families at a loss.

There is research that shows that people who usually eat a lot of sugar, red meat, and very few vegetables and who drink a lot of alcohol tend to experience flare-ups more frequently and for longer than patients who do not, according to Colleen D. Webb, a registered dietitian/clinical nutritionist at the Jill Roberts Center for Inflammatory Bowel Disease of the Weill Cornell Medical Center in New York.

Even this rule doesn't apply to everyone. Noelia, a biologist and researcher, put her 3-year-old daughter on a strict diet of organic beef, chicken and pork, along with specially prepared unprocessed foods. Her child has shown dramatic improvement. The effect on IBD symptoms of the chemicals found in processed food is another area that has not been adequately studied.

"People tolerate food differently," Webb noted. "We have different genetics and different food sensitivities. That's why we avoid making generalizations about anything having to do with nutrition."

Family Conflicts over CAM

Parents make health decisions for their children based on their own instincts and emotions, which can create its own set of hardships. For example, it is painful to impose a restrictive diet on a child, or to inject an antioxidant enzyme into a child who is too young to understand the purported necessity of the process. Parents understand what they're trying to do. Children may not.

If you are a parent or a spouse, your sense of responsibility for minimizing your loved one's symptoms may lead you to feel that you're taking on a mission. If you and your physician have a difference of opinion about what foods or alternative measures may help, you may be walking into a predicament.

Amy described how hard it was for her son Jesse, who was diagnosed with colitis at 6, to understand why he couldn't eat sugar, which she thought set off his symptoms. "He'd always been able to eat what he wanted and it was hard not to do that," she said. "The other kids would get candy or a soda after his game and when he couldn't have those things, it was tough. It made him very upset."

Amy talked with a social worker at Boston Children's Hospital who told her that diet was one of the major challenges for kids with IBD. "She told me that social eating is their childhood. Going to a birthday party and not being able to eat the cake or the pizza — what do you do, not go to the party? It's hard for them. You want them to be happy and have an easy childhood, not have to confront a hard challenge."

But it didn't matter, because, ultimately, the diets were no match for Jesse's disease. "He had a bad organ that didn't work," Amy said with resignation. Jesse's symptoms were never controlled. At age 8, he underwent a total colectomy. His colon was replaced with a J-pouch. Now he eats whatever he wants.

It is poignant to hear of children struggling to live up to their parents' well-intentioned instructions. Nicole's parents put her on a gluten-free diet for about a year when she was 10. "That was challenging," she said. "I didn't sneak. I was really good about it, but by the end I was so tired of it. I just wanted a hamburger. I told them I hated the diet, didn't feel it was doing anything for me, except I was cranky. They saw it wasn't really doing much so they let it slide."

Carol and her daughter, Gina, have a complicated relationship around diet. Carol is a small, intense, fast-talking woman who is disciplined about what she eats and fiercely focused on her daughter's wellbeing. She was plagued by doubts about Gina's diagnosis of Crohn's disease in middle school: Did her daughter really suffer from Crohn's at all? Maybe it was just a reaction to the medications prescribed for Crohn's. Could it be lactose intolerance misdiagnosed as Crohn's? Did the lactose in the Pentaza she was prescribed cause a flare-up in her disease?

Virtually every time Gina's disease flared, Carol pressed her to follow different diets to control her symptoms. Among the diets were those outlined in several books, including *Breaking the Vicious Cycle: The Specific Carbohydrate Diet* by Elaine Gottschall, which advocates gluten-, dairy- and sugar-free foods, and *The Hallelujah Diet: Experience the Optimal Health You Were Meant to Have*, by George Malkmus and Peter Shockey, which advocates a diet made up mostly of raw foods. Another diet recommended drinking only carrot juice.

Gina vacillated between appreciating her mother's vigilance and resenting it. She credits her mother's focus on healthy foods with her relative wellbeing, noting that she never had to undergo surgery, unlike many of her friends with Crohn's. But the tug of war between them over the years took a psychological toll on them both.

"She was on a juicing kick," said Gina, referring to the time her mother decided that carrot juice was the answer to Gina's Crohn's. "It's easily absorbed in the system," Carol explained to me. "We'd buy 25 pounds of organic carrots and apples. Absolutely delicious." Despite Carol's zealous faith in the new approach, the experiment did not end well.

"She was force-feeding me carrot juice," Gina recalled. "My stomach still hurt and I still had to go to the bathroom. So I locked myself in the bathroom. She tried to unscrew the doorknob to open the door because she would not leave until I drank the carrot juice. I stayed in the bathroom with the door locked until she left for work. I refused."

Carol, defending herself, said: "She didn't tell me at the time that she felt the carrot juice was giving her diarrhea. She was just saying, 'No, I'm not doing it.' I'd say 'Yes, you have to do this.'" Carol later apologized to her daughter. "She was sorry," Gina recalled. "That was a tough day. You felt the desperation on both sides: me wanting to be better and her trying to find something that works."

Children who are sick look to their parents to make them feel better. And when their parent turns to alternative therapies, children follow. Only later are they able to reflect on the effect the alternative therapies had on them, for better or worse.

Nicole was diagnosed at 10, so her parents were making all the decisions about her medical care. Her first physician prescribed more medicine than they were comfortable with, so they sent Nicole to a doctor who practiced holistic medicine. "I got injections of glutathione," she said. "I really don't know what it did. It was supposed to help, but it smelled like old people." Her parents sent her to another such doctor. "He had me on amber-root pills you put under your tongue. He had me doing exercises where he'd ring a bell and I'd have talk about what I liked and didn't like about the colitis. That was a very unproductive stage of my life. I was a few years into colitis and my parents were desperately trying to find something that worked that wasn't medicine or surgery."

Clinton was 11 when he was diagnosed with Crohn's. He also complied when his mother, Wendy, tried to find alternative measures. They paid a visit to the Dr. Jonn Matsen, author of *Eating Alive: Prevention Thru Good Digestion*, and followed his program. That didn't work, so Wendy put Clinton on the diet advised by Jordon Rubin, author of *The Maker's Diet: The 40-Day Health Experience That Will Change Your Life Forever*. Rubin claimed that the diet had helped him to conquer his own Crohn's. Clinton was allowed no wheat and no dairy. His mother cooked with rice milk and high-protein hemp seeds.

Along with dietary approaches, Wendy, ever vigilant and hopeful, immediately took Clinton to a naturopath, who prescribed a host of vitamins that supposedly could be absorbed when his body was rejecting anything else he had ingested. "We tried anything," Clinton recalled. "He prescribed herbs. We figured, might as well give it a shot. When medicine's not working, there are other things to try."

As Clinton kept getting sicker and sicker, the naturopath realized his case was more serious than she had the ability to affect. "But she didn't straight up admit it," Clinton said. Wendy took Clinton to a Chinese doctor, who prescribed shark fin cartilage (a substance that is not recommended for children and that has not been shown to have any effectiveness in the treatment of IBD). "We still have it sitting there on the shelf," Clinton said. Clinton became so ill that he was confined to the hospital for two months. His doctors commented that he had really expensive urine because all those supplements had gone right through him.

Clinton decided he wanted to go on conventional medications, despite Wendy's desires. "I didn't want him to go on Humira because of the side effects," she said. She added that she had told him flatly, "You're not going on the medicine." But, she said, "He looked at me and said, 'Mom, it's my decision.' He was 16. I was devastated. I knew he was tired of being sick and wanted to be a normal teenager." She began to weep. "It was a pretty ugly time."

Clinton "was a good sport for a while," Wendy said, but he kept getting more ill, more discouraged, and more depressed. Finally, his colon had to be removed and he has worn an ostomy bag ever since.

Alisa's expedition into CAM is a chronicle of determination, persistence, and, most of all, her desire to ease her symptoms from ulcerative colitis. At one time or another, she visited a chiropractor three times a week, an acupuncturist and a Chinese healer — all without a positive result. She tried eating with the seasons, practicing yoga, and drinking liquid chlorophyll, all to no avail, and she experimented with probiotic herbs, which, she said, were helpful for about five days and then the colitis came back. Hoping for serenity and insight, Alisa focused on yoga and meditation, "shifting my perspective on colitis, trying to listen to what it's trying to tell me."

CAM Is Everywhere

Gastroenterologists recognize that CAM is part of the landscape for about half their patients, and most of these specialists have no objection when patients seek untraditional treatments, as long as the treatments don't conflict with conventional medical therapies.

For example, for about four years before I was told that my entire colon had to be removed, I went to an acupuncturist. Right before my colectomy, I asked my surgeon if he objected to my taking a Chinese herbal pill my acupuncturist had told me would speed up the healing process post-surgery. To my surprise, my surgeon had no objection. I perceived my healing to be fast and smooth, which I, of course, attributed to the tiny pill and a post-surgical acupuncture treatment. I felt almost smug that I had avoided a painful and lengthy recovery period, even as I grudgingly had to admit that I had no proof that the pill and acupuncture had had anything to do with it.

Indeed, alternative measures have not been adequately studied. "While scientific evidence exists regarding some CAM therapies," states the CCFA on its website (www.ccfa.org), "for the most part, well-designed scientific studies to answer questions such as whether these therapies are safe and whether they work for the purposes for which they are used have not been conducted."

Therefore, many doctors are reluctant to recommend CAM therapies in the absence of proven statistical information. One physician challenges the CCFA position. "Dismissing the entire group as 'quack medicine' may be a disservice to patients and families searching for additional ways to manage their disease," writes Dr. Christopher Jolley, associate professor of pediatrics and chief of pediatric gastroenterology at the University of Florida College of Medicine, Gainesville.

"It can strain trust and may result in poorer patient–physician communication," He writes. He also dryly notes the following: "Several of the more conventional therapies for IBD have limited data supporting them, particularly in the pediatric population. Pediatric use of drugs, including some with proven toxicity, frequently is extrapolated from adult data, which is hardly pristine scientific medical practice."(Frei, 2009)

Emotional Healing

It is hard not to take IBD personally. It is hard not to ask, "Why is this happening to me? What did I do to make this happen?" Patients understand that their high emotions did not cause their disease, but, at times, their anger and helplessness on top of their symptoms make life seem unbearable. Like any chronic illness or cancer, IBD can bring up self-pity, self-blame, and confusion. How to get out of this and move on with life is another way to take control.

"Living with inflammatory bowel disease is an emotional rollercoaster," wrote Marisa, in the blog she wrote at 26 after being diagnosed at 13 with ulcerative colitis. "You have no idea how long the good days will last. It is an enormous amount of trial and error with medications, food and just lifestyle choices in general. The amount of missed events and special occasions is far too plentiful in the life of an IBD patient. The lack of control can leave you feeling helpless and frustrated. The anger and feelings of frustration when nothing seems to be going right are all too common."

Marisa, who has undergone 14 major surgeries, recommends that patients connect with a therapist or therapy group and particularly with a group of other people with IBD, "because if you let the emotional part get out of hand, pretty soon you're years into it and extremely overwhelmed and it's a lot more difficult to deal with. The emotional thing is huge."

You don't have to suffer the extremes of IBD to feel emotional pain from it. I spent years in psychotherapy, trying to fathom what my colon was trying to tell me. Ultimately, I understood that the flare-ups of my colitis were, so to speak, sending up a flare to alert me that I was repressing anger and despair in an attempt to seem like a normal teenager and young adult. It happened that my colon was my genetic weak spot and all the stress and unhappiness of my life were attacking the vulnerable organ in my body. That's how I thought about it.

What this monumental insight did for my colon is unclear. After years of inflammation but no symptoms, I still ended up with precancerous cells and the need for a total colectomy, but in the interim, my insight made me happier and better adjusted. My colitis shadowed my life, but it was no longer an all- consuming preoccupation.

It may seem improbable to try to extract meaning from your IBD to deepen your understanding of yourself. Obviously, this is not something a young child can tackle, but, at whatever age, finding meaning in your IBD can comfort you, place your experience in context, and remove shame and blame.

Alisa experienced something akin to this after being pregnant for two weeks before miscarrying. During those two weeks, she had no colitis symptoms. The experience of the pregnancy and the lack of symptoms were strongly emotional for her. She started seeing a therapist to deal with her shame and guilt. "I'm a Catholic," she explained, "so I was trying to address what came out as toxicity in my colon."

The notion that you can become better than you were before your illness seems like a too-far-distant shore. But it can happen. Rebeka said she had made it to that shore because of all the meditation and yoga she practiced. "I don't get stressed out, and it's made me a more balanced person, for sure," she said. Before her diagnosis with ulcerative colitis, she said, "I didn't want to be stressed out and neurotic, but I wasn't making any efforts to change." However, there is nothing like seeing more blood than stool in a toilet bowl or suffering stabbing pains in your stomach to motivate you to think about what might help to stabilize your mind and spirit, if not your bowels.

Until patients find a path to make peace with their diseased digestive system, they will continue to wage an internal emotional and psychological battle, observed Joel. Joel has had a few of those battles himself after being diagnosed with ulcerative colitis in his late 20s while he worked as an engineer for a multi-million dollar government program. "A lot of people hate what they're dealing with," he said. "They hate their body. They hate themselves. They hate other people." Joel left the corporate world to heal himself. He went to nutrition school and became a yoga teacher. What that taught him, he said, was "that you have to love what you have and deal with it from that point." This is easier said than done, but certainly something to aspire to.

Conclusion

Finding a single CAM approach that will consistently alleviate IBD would be, as they say, awesome. Unfortunately, that is as unlikely as finding a single magic bullet to cure the disease, although researchers hope one day that will occur. Until then, there is no evidence — scientific or anecdotal —that any single alternative approach works for everyone. In short, every person must figure out what treatments work for them, another frustrating chink in the confusing world of IBD.

CHAPTER EIGHT
Urgency

When IBD patients are on the brink of losing control and running to find a bathroom, they naturally want to somehow maintain their dignity and equanimity. These attributes, in the moment, are not easy to access.

Because of inflammation near the rectum, patients feel in constant need to pass stool, whether the colon is empty or not. When you're trying to live a life as normally as possible despite having IBD, there's almost nothing as infantilizing or demeaning as losing control of your bowels in public or while alone in your car.

Urgency dominates the lives of about 30 percent of people with IBD, limiting their activities and getting in the way of school and work. Urgency, or tenesmus, as it's technically called, usually affects people with ulcerative colitis, but it can also occur when Crohn's disease is located in the large intestine.

April, a 28-year-old teacher, describes a classic case of tenesmus. "It got to the point where I was probably having a sort of bowel movement maybe 40 times a day and I'd feel like I couldn't hold it," she said, the memory gushing out. "It was mucuous-y tissue coming out. It was so awful. I would have blood in my underwear and the stools that were pencil thin. Then I felt like I had to keep going, but nothing was coming out but blood and tissue."

Because urgency is such a frequent side effect of IBD, it is surprising to find so little guidance either online or in academic papers to help people deal with it socially and emotionally. Perhaps this speaks to the complexity of feelings that arise: helplessness, despair, shame, panic, and loneliness.

The intensity of the feelings that accompany urgency make it unlikely that people who experience it will forget the circumstances. This is certainly true of my accidents. Decades later, I have a vivid memory of briskly walking home from work in the midst of a colitis flare-up, and realizing that I would not make it to my apartment in time. The cramps were so intense that I doubted I could hold it in for ten more seconds, much less the ten more minutes it would take to get home. I darted into a chain restaurant and dashed to the bathroom just to the left of the front door.

I lost control as soon as I entered the restroom. Bloody diarrhea spread across the floor. Mortified, I quickly hid in a bathroom stall when I heard someone enter behind me. "Oh my God," she yelled. I cringed. There was nothing I could do. I felt awful for being the cause of this stranger's distress. I also felt humiliated, because here I was, a fully grown woman, cowering in a bathroom stall just having haplessly failed potty training. After she left abruptly, I tiptoed through the mess, got a wad of paper towels and tried to mop up the floor, but there was far too much to do a thorough scrubbing. Sad to say, I fled, too ashamed to notify a staff person that a cleanup was needed in the women's restroom.

Once an accident happens, the possibility of future accidents makes patients acutely worried and self-conscious. Even if an accident has never actually occurred, the fear that it might can be paralyzing. Fear begins to rule over daily life.

"A lot of people never had an accident but are scared of having one," said Dr. Laura C. Reigada, a psychologist and an adjunct assistant professor of pediatrics at the Mount Sinai School of Medicine in New York. With her colleagues, she interviewed 200 patients for studies on anxiety and IBD. (Reigada, 2011, 2013, 2014) "Most kids and young adults can find a bathroom when they're having urgency, but fear often controls their lives," she said. "In their minds, an accident is the worst thing ever and they hold onto that very strongly.

"The unpredictability of urgency means kids have a lot of anxiety about it," she continued, "especially in a school setting," when "they're already at an elevated stage of vulnerability and anxiety." Concerned that classmates will notice how often they get up from their desk to use the bathroom, students try to disguise their visits to the bathroom, sometimes by asking to see the school nurse and instead using the toilet.

Adina, 27, proves this point. If she had to go to the bathroom more than once in an hour in high school, she felt embarrassed. "Most teachers look at you funny," she said. "I'd say, 'I really need a drink of water,' or, 'I need to go to the nurse's office.'"

Often, patients with urgency seek advice from their gastroenterologist, but, Dr. Reigada said, "Doctors don't usually treat their emotional issues, and patients don't realize it can be treated with psychological interventions." She said she wishes more children and young adults would seek the assistance of social workers and psychologists to help them cope.

The anxiety of living with and anticipating urgency occurs in many settings. From things as ordinary as taking a morning run or riding in a car to a momentous event like walking down the aisle at one's own wedding, urgency and its attendant anxiety turn situations into a huge risk.

Before her wedding, Adina's biggest fear was that she would have to leave the *chuppah* (the Jewish bridal canopy) to run to the bathroom. This is not the usual concern for brides. As it turned out, she got through the wedding without incident.

As an antidote to their fears of possible accidents, patients prepare themselves. "In my purse, in case I start feeling really bad, I carry adult diapers," said Adina, who once had to get off a horse and go behind a tree. Nerissa, 25, says she "still gets nervous about going out and I have to prepare myself with hand sanitizer, panties, and wipes." Nerissa has never actually lost control outside of a bathroom.

Children depend on their parents to get them out of a fix. When he was 8, Josh was playing with his ice hockey team when he skated to the edge of the rink and whispered to his mother, "I got to get off the rink, and I got to go to the bathroom." His mother, Jacque, threw him over her shoulder, thrust him into her car and drove to the first restaurant she could find. "He's in full gear," she recalled. "I tore it off piece by piece, hoping I didn't let him lose his dignity."

After that incident, Jacque prepared for the next time. "We had a bag of plastic liners, a change of clothes, and a children's portable training potty in the car. He had somewhere to go and a blanket to make it as private as possible. You'd be surprised at how many public places won't let you use their bathroom or don't have one."

"Be prepared" is the most practical advice that Dr. Reigada and the CCFA have for people worried about urgency. The CCFA recommends that people who suffer urgency and who are traveling by car choose roads with the most bathrooms, probably not the most scenic routes. They recommend bringing their own toilet paper, soothing wipes, ointments, change of underwear, extra clothes and a small bottle of hand sanitizer that can go through airport security when necessary.

This is useful advice, but unfortunately it does not work for everybody and it doesn't address the emotional charge that tenesmus inflicts.

Even when people are well prepared and they know the exact layout of the bathrooms, accidents can happen. LoriAnn, who was diagnosed with colitis at 21, lived near Disney World, and she and her husband held season passes to the park. "I know the bathrooms like the back of my hand," she said. "I'd have to go to the bathroom every two seconds. A couple of times, I didn't even make it to the bathroom and lost it in front of everybody. I went all over myself. It stops me from going out with my friends," she continued. "I can't go to the beach because there's no bathroom. A lot of my friends don't understand. They ask me, 'Can't you just come?'"

Sports

For young people with IBD who love playing sports, urgency either shuts them down or, at the very least, impedes the activities that keep them athletically engaged, whether it's playing ice hockey, rowing, running, or playing golf.

For example, Jason, diagnosed at 22, projects the strong image of the football and basketball player that he was in college. But in his first full-time job, he lost 50 pounds in six months and had to go to the bathroom 20 times a day. "I'd take a bite out of my sandwich at lunch and have to go to the bathroom," he said. "Blood — the whole nine yards."

A series of tests showed that Jason had moderate-to-severe pan colitis, meaning that IBD affected his entire colon. Now, he plans his activities around his flare-ups. "If I want to go out for a run, a lot of times I won't, because I get scared I'll have to go," he said. "Yesterday, my wife had to pick me up. When I'm not in a flare, I feel like a normal person. I have energy. But whenever I do something too intense, I start having blood in my stool." Jason's urgency has gotten worse. Playing golf one day, he had an accident while he was with his dad and friends.

Laura, an attorney, panics when she goes shopping, takes a long walk, or goes on a run and there is no bathroom nearby or she fears there won't be. In a pinch, she runs home or uses "really disgusting Porta-Pottys in parks." She is adept at begging restaurant employees to use their bathroom. For a long time, she didn't run outside, "because it was such a scary thing. Instead, I'd run on a treadmill." Laura had such anxiety that she was put on an antidepressant. She has never had an accident, yet the apprehension that it might happen reigns over her life.

Traveling

Planes present problems for people with urgency because of the regulations that passengers stay in their seats during takeoff, landing, and turbulence. Long lines for the bathroom on a plane also create great anxiety for anyone with urgency. Adina carries a CCFA card that says, "I Can't Wait," and she hands it to the stewardess during takeoff. "When they say you can't get up," she said, "I've told the stewardesses I have to go to the bathroom." It works.

Stefanie, diagnosed with ulcerative colitis at 26, sits in her airplane seat during takeoff and manages with great effort to keep control of her bowels. Getting onto her father's boat was another matter. "My dad had a small motor boat, and I stopped going out in it because it didn't have a bathroom," Stefanie said. "Most of the time, you can pee in the water, but other things you can't do."

Being in a car for any length of time is one of the scariest places for someone with IBD to be when urgency hits. Some patients solve the problem by not leaving their house. "I didn't want to go anywhere," said Aaron, who was diagnosed at 18. "I'd have to go 15 to 20 times a day. Everything I ate went right through me. I didn't enjoy going out because I was afraid of not getting to the bathroom in time. I'd have to go in my pants while I was driving. It was horrible."

Working

Dr. Reigada, the psychologist, says young working adults use the same concealment techniques that children use in school. They worry that their co-workers will notice their frequent comings and goings, and they "will do all kinds of things to mask that they're going to the bathroom," she said. "They go in a different direction" and then circle back to the bathroom.

Other workers try to adhere to their workplace rules so as not to stand out. April was in her first year of teaching, and urgency took her concentration away from her students and kept her in constant discomfort. "You have students —you can't just leave," she said. "I seriously thought I might go on disability. During classroom breaks, I would walk down the hall as quickly as I could, because as much as I wanted to run, you're not supposed to run on campus. You need to be a role model."

Jill, diagnosed at age 7, worked as a waitress while she was in graduate school. "It got to the point where it was interfering with my job," she said of her urgency. "I'd have to go to the bathroom a lot and I had three tables I was responsible for, and I'd have bleeding and leakage while I was walking around."

Lori Ann finds mornings to be the worst time for her urgency. "I go five times from the time I get up to the time I go to work," she said. "I might be late to work because I have to stop at McDonald's, a 7-Eleven, anywhere that has a bathroom at 7 a.m. Because if I don't go right that second, I'm not going to make it to work."

Maureen, diagnosed at 15, described her life and, in fact, the lives of everyone with urgency as "bathroom-centric all the time." After college, she took the subway every day to her first job. She had to get off the train four or five times to go to the bathroom.

Restroom Access Act

Stephanie tried to use a bathroom in retail stores several times, but she was refused. "They don't understand," she said. "I ended up having an accident on the streets of Philadelphia. That was the only time I actually s—- myself in public. I understand there are cards you can get at this point to give to people."

There are, indeed, cards to gain access to restrooms, but there is no guarantee they will work. The effectiveness of "I Can't Wait" cards issued by the CCFA depends on the kindness and responsiveness of the store staff. But there is a law in several states that doesn't leave things to chance. The Restroom Access Act requires businesses to open their employee-only restrooms to people who can prove they have IBD. The law, first passed by Illinois in 2005, allows access to an employees-only restroom to anyone with a medical condition.

As of this writing, 13 states have joined in: Colorado, Connecticut, Illinois, Kentucky, Massachusetts, Michigan, Minnesota, Ohio, Oregon, Tennessee, Texas, Wisconsin and Washington. The law's genesis was a shopping trip to an Old Navy store by 14-year-old Ally Bain, who had been diagnosed with Crohn's disease at the age of 11. Ally needed to find a restroom quickly, but the store manager refused to let her use the employee-only bathroom, so she couldn't help but soil herself. Ally and her mother successfully lobbied for a law requiring businesses to grant access if someone can show they have IBD.

In his blog, Empowered by Kids, Justin Vandergrift, whose daughter has ulcerative colitis, points out that just walking into a store and requesting access to a restroom does not guarantee you'll get it, regardless of any law. Many employees may not know about the law. "In the end," he writes, "you are still dealing with a human on the other end of your request."

Although they don't address the need to get to a bathroom immediately, there are a couple of resources for people looking for public bathrooms. One is https://www.sitorsquat.com and another is www.thebathroomdiaries.com. There are also apps. You can find them on: http://www.everydayhealth.com/crohns-disease-pictures/five-apps-to-help-you-find-a-bathroom.aspx#03

Coping

Urgency doesn't always have to truncate activities. Some of the people I interviewed seemed to deal with their tenesmus through sheer will. Michal tenaciously back-packed through Europe after college graduation, even though she frequently had to run to the bathroom and was getting sicker and sicker. In Belgium, she couldn't take it anymore. She went to a doctor, who immediately diagnosed ulcerative colitis. "I was 23, you know. I wanted to keep backpacking. I'd just run around trying to find a bathroom. *This is crazy*, I thought. *Maybe I should go home. No, I'm having such fun. I don't want to leave.* I stayed in urban areas. I'd run into cafes. If I went to a museum, I'd figure out the layout of the museum and where the bathrooms were." Michal backpacked through France, Belgium, Holland, Germany, Prague, Greece, and Israel. The doctor gave her supposito-ries, which minimized the bleeding and urgency. "I had to be kind of creative," she said. "I never had an accident."

Some people manage their emotional response by keep-ing at the front of their mind an awareness of the reasons for their urgency. Nobody teaches this, although psy-chotherapy may help to foster it. By accepting urgency as a fact of your life, you can de-fang it and render it less threat-ening. Just as you accept IBD as the new normal, you can accept urgency as your new normal and take all the medic-inal and emotional steps you can to alleviate it. What you accept can't attack you.

Bob was a teenager at the wheel when he realized he wouldn't make it home. Thinking quickly, he parked his car next to the shoulder on the highway and ran into the woods to evacuate. "I didn't wipe it all, just went home, stripped down, showered and told my mom what happened. I was fine. I was very cognizant about what was going on with my body."

Nerissa doesn't minimize the panic and anxiety that built up inside her as urgency escalated. However, speaking from a more relaxed perspective while in remission, she said she concentrates on trying to stay calm and fixates on dissolving her stress and tension. "I don't let it all go to my stomach," she said. "I just make sure I know where every toilet is."

Tiffany is a tough young woman who takes a practical approach to her colitis. She deals with her urgency by refusing to let it tell her what she can't do. She participates in the most improbable activity for someone with urgency: re-enactments of medieval battles, which require her to don armor, preventing her, to put it mildly, from easily using a toilet.

"If I think I'm going to be away from a bathroom for a very long time," she said, "I take an over-the-counter anti-diarrheal preventively. It makes me pretty nauseous the next day when I go off of it. In the summer, I get into armor and I'm away from a bathroom for five hours. I take it in the morning before I get into the armor. My doctor thinks it's awesome."

Internet chat rooms reveal that an anti-diarrheal is a remedy used by many people with urgency, with varying success. Others try medicinal suppositories, which also work with varying success.

As someone who has experienced urgency, I have a deep understanding for the emotional charge it carries. My fervent wish would be to hand over a remedy to relieve the stress, the worry, and the embarrassment. But, as with all things related to IBD, no single approach works for everyone. I hope that somehow, people with urgency will feel confident enough one day to don a proverbial suit of armor and head into battle to conquer — and accept — their urgency in a way that works for them.

CHAPTER NINE

Depression and Anxiety with IBD

I'll never forget coming into her bedroom and her saying to me, "Who would ever want to marry me?" She was 8 years old. That always rang in my head. I tried to make sure I treated her mind, not just her body.

— **Rebecca,**
speaking about her daughter, Hannah

An 8-year-old with Crohn's disease feels so stripped of her identity as a healthy young girl that she worries she will be unmarriageable when she grows up. Hannah is a haunting example of how Crohn's disease and ulcerative colitis interfere with the way many young people think about themselves and their prospects in life and how much they live with depression and anxiety.

"The diagnosis of a chronic illness such as IBD during childhood can involve a grieving process that begins with shock and disbelief and proceeds through feelings of anguish (sadness) and protest (anger) while [children] assimilate the facts of their condition and adjust to the implications of the disease," write researchers in the journal *Pediatrics*. (Mackner, 2003)

With flaring IBD, simple activities that used to provide pleasure, like eating what you like, playing sports, or running, among many others, are not possible anymore. You feel sick to your stomach when you eat and the foods you eat are restricted. You are chronically fatigued. You run to the bathroom with embarrassing frequency. Your growth and puberty may be delayed and you may have fecal incontinence or steroid-induced weight gain.

However, many young people manage to cope with IBD without damage to their mental health. With milder versions of the disease, it is easier to incorporate IBD into your life. Alex took a positive view of his diagnosis and was thriving in college despite being diagnosed with Crohn's disease. "I accepted that I will have Crohn's probably for the rest of my life," he said. "I'll take pills. It's become part of who I am. I recognize how fortunate I am. It hasn't ruined my life. I got on the growth hormone. I grew so much. Things seemed to get better once I was diagnosed rather than spiral downward. It was good I caught it and I was happy."

Nevertheless, more than 50 percent of young people with IBD experience some level of depression, compared with 9 percent of healthy young people. (Engstrom, 1999)

Reasons for Depression and Anxiety

As has been discussed briefly, anxiety is a pervasive part of the experience of IBD, and it is closely linked to depression. There are many reasons for the confluence of IBD with depression and anxiety. Although many chronic illnesses, such as asthma, diabetes, arthritis, and heart disease are linked to depression and anxiety, IBD has the dubious distinction of being the disease with the highest association with depression and anxiety among young people.

There may be scientific reasons for this that are only now coming to light. The human gut is often referred to as the body's "second brain." It is the only organ to boast its own independent nervous system, an intricate network of

100 million neurons embedded in the gut wall. When you consider the gut's multifaceted ability to communicate with the brain, along with its crucial role in defending the body against the perils of the outside world, "it's almost unthinkable that the gut is not playing a critical role in mind states," said gastroenterologist Dr. Emeran Mayer, director of the Gail and Gerald Oppenheimer Family Center for Neurobiology of Stress at the University of California, Los Angeles. (Carpenter, 2012)

Environmental triggers also link IBD with depression. After a period of adapting to the role of a sick person, for example, young people with diabetes realize that the disease is socially acceptable and it gives no cause for shame. Not so with IBD. The symptoms of IBD are often socially embarrassing, and they are difficult to discuss with peers. This combination of repressed emotions and shame is a perfect recipe for depression, anxiety and stress.

Lori Ann had crying jags after being diagnosed with ulcerative colitis at 21. "Emotionally, I was shot," she recalled. "I couldn't talk to anybody about it. I couldn't understand why a perfectly healthy person could no longer even be able to live a full day normally."

She became particularly depressed after asking her gastroenterologist whether she could bear children. He said possibly not, "Because I can't keep weight on enough to nourish a kid," she said. "I didn't want to accept the fact that I wouldn't be able to have kids. I even told my husband I'd understand if he wanted to leave me, because I can't have kids." (He didn't.) Lori Ann found a sympathetic ear in her pastor's wife, who provided a space for Lori to vent her anger and frustration. "If it weren't for her," she said, "I'd probably be dealing with a lot more depression."

According to psychiatrist Dr. Eva Szigethy and her colleagues at the University of Pittsburgh, who have written extensively on depression and IBD, there is a laundry list of other reasons that IBD can foster depression, among them the loss of independence, the sense of control, privacy, a healthy body image, peer relationships, former roles inside and outside the family, self-confidence and self-esteem, productivity, future plans, familiar daily routines, ways of expressing sexuality, and a pain-free existence. (Szigethy, 2011)

In addition, you may feel guilty for being a burden to your parents. You may have separation anxiety when your parent leaves you for even a short while. You may fear losing love and approval. The resulting reaction is frustration, anger, depression and anxiety.

And it gets worse for those of you who undergo multiple surgeries and hospitalizations. You may also experience post-traumatic stress disorder (PTSD), which is often suffered by soldiers after battle. Young people with IBD fight their own battles, and their mental health is often collateral damage.

It is easy to lose perspective when you have been told that you have an incurable condition and your symptoms are not yet under control. In the midst of your distress, you may think it will always be this bad. This is what Alyssa faced when told she had Crohn's disease. "I had a lot of anxiety because I didn't see remission," she said. "It was extremely overwhelming. If it was this violent the whole time, I didn't want to handle it. I got really depressed and I dealt with [depression] a long time. At age 14, all you want to be is normal and I was far from normal at that point. I was having suicidal thoughts and really felt like, if that was how I was going to be alive, then it really wasn't worth it."

Alyssa's family noticed a strong decline four months into her disease. She had stopped eating. About nine months after she was diagnosed with Crohn's, she was prescribed antidepressants and, after a lengthy search for the right person, she started seeing a psychiatrist twice a week. He diagnosed PTSD and severe depression. The medication kicked in and she began to feel better after six months. More than a decade later, Alyssa still takes medication to treat mild depression and anxiety.

When depression hits, its effects can be almost as pronounced as the physical effects of an IBD flare-up. In the midst of a flare-up, Nerissa, 25, was struck with a sudden bout of depression and what she calls "a little bit of a mental breakdown." She is a professional journalist who was diagnosed with Crohn's disease at age 13, but when she became depressed, she not only couldn't write an article, she couldn't write her name in longhand.

"It was really strange," she said. "Depression attacks you both mentally and physically. I'm a practical person, but I couldn't work. My mind went kaput. I stopped believing in what I was doing. You just have to decide if your job is worth your health or if it's time to move on. I chose to resign from my workplace." For a month, Nerissa stayed with her parents, in a bad state and in retreat from her life. She has since recovered, both from that flare-up of Crohn's and her depression.

Many children ask the "Why me?" question about their enduring embarrassment and pain from IBD. "Why do I have to have this pain? Why do I have to be the smallest and weakest in the class?" Shawn asked. "I didn't understand why." Not only young children struggle with this question. Lori Ann was 21 when she asked after being diagnosed with ulcerative colitis, "Was I being punished for something I did? I had been healthy. I couldn't come to terms with it." Gillian, 30, asks and answers. "I asked 'Why me?' all the time. At this point, it *is* me. I've got to deal with it. Having my daughter as a driving force keeps me going."

"'Poor me' is what you read between the lines," said Dr. Kodman-Jones, the psychologist who worked until 2011 with children with IBD at the Children's Hospital of Philadelphia. "It's a process of helping the kid understand that this is a lot more complex than a week and a half flu, where, when you sleep, you get better. It's not like anything they've experienced before. Kids have to build in a level of emotional complexity in thinking that wasn't there before." In a hospital setting, she added, GI nurses address children's existential questions. "What did I do wrong?" "You did nothing wrong." "Why didn't my brother get sick?" "Your body's different. You may be a fantastic reader and he isn't. You're more sensitive in this way."

Some young people blame themselves for their IBD, thinking that their illness is a punishment for something they did wrong. "There were times Trinity would say, 'Why is this happening to me? Is it something I did, because I was mean to my sister the day before? I'll fix it,' her mother, LeAnne, recalled. LeAnne found it difficult to explain to Trinity, who was diagnosed at age 8 and who had had symptoms from age 2, that there was no reason for her getting the disease. The randomness of it was inexplicable.

Dr. Kodman-Jones has observed the phenomenon of self-blame and IBD. "It's confusing, especially in the first flare. Young people feel typically pretty healthy until the flare. It's all new. They can't wrap their minds around why they're so sick," she said. "After the first flare has resolved, for the most part, they almost have this feeling that it's never going to come back. They forget about it. The second flare is when they really see that it's a chronic illness. Then they really feel punished. They must be bad because it's come back. It's the second flare they mourn the most about their condition."

Clinton, a teenager diagnosed with severe Crohn's disease who underwent surgery, said, "I've known some patients who become very depressed and, even if they're well enough to resume daily life, they can't and don't. A couple of years after, it's sad to see people let IBD overcome who they are. It's a part of me, but not who I am."

Medication-induced Depression

The symptoms of IBD are not alone in producing depression and anxiety. Some IBD medication can also create mental repercussions, particularly Prednisone, which is known for causing mood swings. (See Chapter Five on medications). But because the extreme emotions feel so real, it can be hard to relate them to your medication.

Jonathan was tapering off Prednisone. He was in graduate school, studying in a program he loved, when one morning he awoke feeling utterly bleak. "All of a sudden I go into a tailspin depression," he said. "I'd never experienced depression before. I'm in no upheaval with personal relationships or in conflict with my family. Darkness. All of a sudden, I could not get motivated. I couldn't go to the store to buy toothpaste- — scary stuff I'd never experienced before. It took two weeks to bring it up with my parents."

Jonathan's parents sent him to a counseling center where he received short-term therapy. It didn't help. Nobody there asked Jonathan what medication he was taking. He thought about dropping out of his academic program. He stopped going to class, because he couldn't face the world outside his apartment. His parents considered hospitalizing him.

One morning, he forced himself out of bed and went on a run and "saw light coming out of the sky for the first time." He resumed going to class. Feeling rejuvenated, he quoted a popular psychologist of the time to a good friend, telling her, "'Death is your friend. You don't have all the time in the world. Let people know how you feel.'" "For me, it was a profound thought about how to come out of my depression," he said. "She heard the word 'death' and freaked out."

The friend immediately dropped him off at a clinic to see a psychiatrist. The first thing the doctor asked was whether Jonathan was on any medications. "I tell him about the Crohn's and Prednisone," Jonathan said. "He's like, 'Bingo.' It's the first time I heard this could happen. Depression is a side effect of Prednisone."

Post-Traumatic Stress Disorder

Post-Traumatic Stress Disorder (PTSD) is associated with severe trauma, such as abuse, violence, or battle. It is often seen in soldiers returning from war with serious mental disorders caused by what they've seen and done. PTSD is an anxiety disorder in which you feel out of control and often terrified. It's not uncommon for counselors to diagnose seriously ill patients with PTSD attributed to prolonged hospitalizations and repeated surgeries. One study found that one in five patients with Crohn's disease suffers from PTSD. (Camara, 2010)

Marisa's PTSD, anxiety, and depression were so severe, she wanted her life to end. Long hospitalizations and 14 major surgeries took a severe toll on her mental health. "All these surgeries gave me very bad nightmares and flashbacks from being in the hospital so much," she said.

Marisa is voluble about her mental pain. During her hospitalizations, she said, "There were a lot of times when the emotional pain was so unbelievable, I really did not even want to make it through the next day. I really just wanted some idiot resident to overmedicate me so I didn't have to feel the reality of life anymore. The physical pain was a relief in a lot of ways, because it stopped me from thinking. It became the only focus. When I was in agony, I couldn't think about how I just had been sliced open, was hooked up to a million machines and tubes, was unable to go home and felt like a prisoner."

Dr. Kodman-Jones and other psychologists I interviewed understand the possible connection between PTSD and IBD, but they are cautious about making the diagnosis. "I can see where it's possible," Kodman-Jones said. "I wouldn't totally rule it out. Multiple hospitalizations are pretty scary to kids. If you're not getting better, you do develop the thinking that there's something wrong with you. Second of all, if they're really sick, a lot of the symptoms like throwing up or having diarrhea keep reoccurring. They could feel traumatized by that. When you feel threatened by the whole process and you feel you're going to die, I would never rule it out." However, she added, "I think it would be more on the rare side than the common side."

Tiffany did not feel depressed when she was focused on her physical pain from Crohn's and a bowel obstruction. Instead, her depression kicked in after surgery, when she felt physically better. "You're no longer holding yourself up, because you don't have to," she said.

This is another phenomenon Dr. Kodman-Jones understands. "You're getting support from the hospital. Then you're better and everybody pulls away and you're left with yourself," she said. "You're now left with all the ramifications of what happened. And if you didn't think about it along the way, it's going to feel like a huge, empty place."

Nevertheless, for most patients, depression rises and falls with their symptoms — the gut-brain connection, as one patient called it. "It's a little bit of a chicken and egg thing," said Anna. "I have depression and anxiety that can precede a flare." On two occasions, once in seventh grade and once in graduate school, she felt depressed and exhausted from trying to hold it together. "I was consumed with anxiety about whether I'd get better and be able to meet the responsibilities I have" and the anxiety coincided with a flare.

"There is a very strong correlation with anxiety and G.I. problems," said Dr. Philip Yucht, a New Jersey-based psychologist, who himself has Crohn's disease. "They're often treated by the same medications, which suggest the pathways may be related. People who suffer from anxiety for a long period of time will ultimately become depressed. It's hard for young people who want to go out and live and be with their friends and have fun, especially when they have significant cases," he said. "One patient was a teenager, about 18, with Crohn's, who was really depressed about it. He would pass gas and leak and didn't know what to do about it. He was ashamed of it. He didn't want to tell anybody. He was really struggling. When you're in that kind of position as a young person, you don't have the wherewithal to manage it."

Nevertheless, as with everything connected with IBD, anxiety and stress do not always coincide with a flare-up of the disease.

Stress and Anxiety

I don't know when I've been more stressed than I was during and shortly after my first marriage. My husband was physically and emotionally abusive. I took my two children — ages 3 years and 8 months — and got out. My parents were dead; I was an only child with relatives living far away. And yet, to my amazement, my colitis remained in remission the entire time. I am sure there are many others who can attest to the irregularity and unpredictability of what triggers their IBD, but most of the people interviewed did not have my experience. Stress is often a trigger for them.

Joel was lead engineer for a multimillion-dollar government program and he left it to reduce his stress and its effects on his ulcerative colitis. He became a yoga teacher and health coach and took a course to increase his skills as a public speaker. Nevertheless, before he goes in front of a roomful of people, he feels the urge to run to the bathroom. "That's how I deal with stress, through my stomach," he said. He has limited expectations that this will ever change.

Stress and anxiety act as the body's alarm system. They deal with threats or tense situations. The body and the mind prepare themselves physically and emotionally to deal with danger. But if the alarm never shuts off, stress and anxiety can become overwhelming and make it hard to carry out your daily routine. Having IBD means that you never know when the next flare might come or what might set it off, making stress and anxiety constant companions. As in Joel's case, your digestive system is ready to act up in stressful situations.

Marisa was beset by severe colitis symptoms and severe anxiety, unaware of the relationship between her emotions and the disease until she saw a video posted online by another young woman with the disease. "I felt so alone when I was experiencing it," she said. "I felt there was something wrong with me for feeling those things. All these unpredictable flare-ups, fatigue, bleeding, and pain are going to cause emotional issues. I got down on myself. It wasn't until I watched videos on anxiety that I thought, 'Oh my God, somebody else has anxiety?' I started doing research. Other people feel these feelings too."

Patients and their families notice the cyclical nature of stress, depression, and the recurrence of symptoms. "It's a cycle," said Adina. "I get stressed out about flaring, worried that I will flare and it causes a flare. I try not to let it."

"You do everything you can," said Dr. Kodman-Jones. "You want to be over it. You can't always be over it. You're doing everything you need to do and you're not getting better. It's pretty devastating."

Isabelle, who was diagnosed with Crohn's at age 15, had been an anxious person before her illness, and IBD created that much more anxiety. "My friends are really supportive, but they sometimes say the wrong thing and I feel isolated and anxious," she said. "And not being able to sleep contributes to anxiety. What's going to come next? When am I going to have another flare? I'm still finding the treatment that works."

Elijah's parents recognized the pattern that stress played in his recurrent Crohn's. During the summers when he was in camp, his Crohn's was quiescent. As soon as he returned home to go to school, the symptoms would reoccur.

In addition to the shame and embarrassment about having IBD, some patients also expressed a reluctance to see a psychotherapist or take psychiatric medication. After coaxing from parents or a spouse, patients often relent and they are later glad they did.

"It was hard to admit I needed help," said Adina, a 27-year-old woman with ulcerative colitis. "My life was stressful, my colitis was getting worse, probably because I was stressed out, and I couldn't get out of that funk. I was fearful of taking something that affects my psyche. I was always fine with talking through things, but never liked the idea of psychological medicine. Now I understand that kind of help is not negative. A therapist put me on anti-anxiety drugs. They really helped. I'm also less fearful. Now if I'm feeling that I'm too high stressed and I can't calm down, I recognize that I can take the pills on an as-needed basis. It's also positive to speak with someone who's not my husband and not a friend about the stresses in my life."

Who Succeeds and Why

Dr. Ingemar Engstrom and his colleagues at the Department of Child and Youth Psychiatry, Uppsala University, Sweden, researched IBD and its effects on young people, and found that children who were resilient both psychologically and socially shared a number of character traits. They came from all walks of life and from families with different income brackets. They had a curiosity about their disease and an eagerness to learn more about it. These children also felt a sense of control. "They thought that they could, in one way or another, affect the course of their disease to a certain extent," he wrote. They could all name stresses in their lives that negatively affected their disease.

In the group with more successful coping skills, "an open, permissive climate within the family with a well-functioning family social network was more common," the researchers found. The young people had someone to talk to about their reactions toward the disease. There was room to exhibit anxiousness, depression, anger, or despair. The listener was sometimes a family member, often the mother, but could in some cases be someone outside the family.

Louie does not fit this profile. He lives alone with his daughter in a small Southern town, far from extended family. Despite the lack of family, he keeps his Crohn's disease at bay with a variety of techniques, one of which is a refusal to give in to depression, stress, and anxiety. "I am a much stronger person mentally, I think, because I've gone through so much illness as a kid. I just know that it's something I have to live with for the rest of my life. For myself and my daughter, I don't give in to the disease. I'll never do that. A lot of people have a tendency to give in, thinking, I'll just be sick my whole life. I don't feel sorry for myself. I'll keep going. I won't let it stop me. I get up and move on."

Gina is also matter-of-fact about her solution to depression. "I've had moments of depression when I'm curled up in a ball," she said. But she has a bucket list of things to look forward to when she feels well enough. "I live my bucket list every day," she said. "I went skydiving. We're planning our next trip."

Psychologist/author Martin Seligman's work on learned optimism points the way toward a healthier approach to IBD. If children take a pessimistic outlook on their illness, they might say, "I am always going to be sick; I am not getting better." Or, "I might feel a little better, but it is going to keep happening." Finally, a child might personalize what has happened and say, 'There is something about me. God does not love me and that is why this is happening to me and not someone else. I am bad."

Individuals who adopt an optimistic perspective might say, "I am sick but it will not last and I will learn what to do to be healthy. If the disease does come back, I will know what to do to improve more quickly." Or, "I might be sick, but I am still a good person and God [or parents, doctors or psychologists] are there to help me with this challenge," thus not personalizing the disease.

Young people with a severe form of IBD can nevertheless find acceptance and a sense of control, and they can stabilize their mental health. "I've struggled with anxiety and depression for a long time," Wendy acknowledged. "Even after my most recent surgery, both really plagued me. When I think about the future, I think about trying to get in as many of the things that I really want to be doing. The things you can do to make yourself happy are so important. There's no reason to do anything that isn't really making you happy. It [Crohn's] is going to come back, but if I dwell on that and wait for that, I'm going to waste everything I can do before it comes back."

CHAPTER TEN

Growing Up with IBD: A Gordian Knot

There were times I'd say, "Why can't you fix this?" I thought
my mom could do everything.

— **Josh, 22, who has Crohn's disease**

Those of you with IBD must confront not only your physical symptoms and the social and psychological repercussions of your illness, but also your parents' emotional response to the disease.

How you navigate the push-pull reactions to your parents' intercession into your daily life with IBD when you desire autonomy may test your relationship or draw you closer — or it may do both at different times. During your childhood and early teens, you may appreciate your parents' reminders to take your medication. You may be grateful that your mother or father communicates with the doctor on your behalf. You may rely on their sense of responsibility, because you may be forgetful or careless when it comes to consistently attending to your IBD.

Your reaction to parental involvement with your illness changes when you get into your late teens and 20s. Many patients, even those in their 20s, find comfort in knowing that their parents will always be there for them and that they can depend on them when they get ill. Others avoid informing their parents about the day-to-day ups and downs of IBD for fear of upsetting them, because anxiety often causes parents to overreact and create drama when the patient seek calmness.

Cara, 23, who was diagnosed at age 12 with Crohn's disease, appreciates her parents' continued involvement in her life with IBD. When she was first diagnosed, she was too young to comprehend what was going on. Her mother asked the doctors all the pertinent questions about Crohn's and its treatments. "I depended on her a lot then, and I think I still do. I don't know if I would say I'm dependent on my parents, but I feel the need to be taken care of. They're definitely the first people I think of."

Cara is typical of the 20-somethings I interviewed, many of whom rely on their parents to help them through tough times with IBD. Curiously, although many patients I interviewed seemed to show delayed emotional independence and continued to rely on their parents to intercede when they got sick, experts in pediatric gastroenterology hold much younger patients to a higher standard of autonomy. The North American Society for Pediatric Gastroenterology, Hepatology and Nutrition (NASPGHAN) provides the following guidelines for what patients between 12 and 18 are expected to know and do about their IBD:

What You're Supposed To Know

From age 12-14, you should be able to describe your GI condition, name your medications, the amount and times you take them, describe the common side effect of your medications, know your doctors' and nurses' names and roles, use and read a thermometer, answer at least one question during a health care visit, manage regular medical tasks at school, call your doctor's office to make or change an appointment, and describe how your GI condition affects you on a daily basis.

When you are 14-17, you should know the names and purposes of the tests that are done, know what can trigger a flare of your disease, know your medical history, know if you need to transition to an adult gastroenterologist, reorder your medications and call your doctor for refills, answer many questions during a health care visit, spend most of your time alone with the doctor during your visit, understand the risk of not following doctors' orders and understand the impact of drugs and alcohol on your condition as well as the impact of IBD on your sexuality.

Past age 17, you should be able to describe what medications you should avoid because they might interact with your IBD medications, visit your doctor alone or choose who you bring with you during a health care visit, be able to tell someone what new legal rights and responsibilities you gained when you turned 18, manage all your medical tasks when you're at school or work, know how to get more information about IBD, book your own appointments, refill prescriptions and contact your medical team, tell someone how long you can be covered under your parents' health insurance plan and what you need to do to maintain coverage for the next two years, and carry your insurance card with you. (NASPGHAN, 2015)

Why That Is Unrealistic

Patients from the age of 12 through the 20s whom I interviewed view many of the tasks above as belonging to their parents' domain. In some cases, parents are happy to take on these duties, not fully trusting that their child will be responsible for their own care. From the patient's point of view, reliance, trust, and dependence on parents arise in part because IBD is so complicated to handle and difficult to talk about with friends outside the family. When you are young, parents are the only people who are exposed to what living with IBD entails. Home is where you find acceptance, no matter how often you run to the bathroom or lie on the couch incapacitated with stomach pain. No one else, until you are married, is as committed to you as are your parents.

But as essential as parents are in the early years of your life with IBD, your developmental changes do mean that even the best-intentioned parent can get irritated when you stand up to them, despite your disease. Ideally, beginning in the teen years, you will evolve toward what psychologists call individuation, meaning that you differentiate, sometimes wrenchingly so, from your original family and create a separate existence. In short, you become more of who you are and less dependent on your parents, and less dependent on their directives about the management of your IBD.

If your parents are supportive and they promote your independence, their oversight can be incredibly helpful, but the debilitating effects of IBD can hamper your psychological and emotional development while you rely on your parents to sustain you.

Needing Parents

Researchers at Queen Silvia Children's Hospital in Gothenburg, Sweden, wrote, "Young people with IBD need help from parents, not only with medication, diet, hospital matters, pain relief and other symptoms, but also in dealing with bloody and mucous-filled stools, urgency, fistulae, fissures and abscesses and rectally administered medication." They continued: "The indispensable [and] ongoing confidence in parents that the condition [requires] probably reinforces the ambivalence that young people feel towards their parents' care. The intimacy involved with bowel activity is not something that can be readily transferred to peers of the same or opposite sex." (Reichenberg, 2007)

Marisa echoes these observations with equal measures of gratitude for her parents and regret. Becoming sick at 13 with ulcerative colitis drew her closer to her parents during her adolescence, when she otherwise might have pulled away to discover herself. "My parents are my heroes," she said directly. "I looked up to them, and they always had the answers."

Nevertheless, her dependence came at a price. Because of the severity of her disease, "I haven't had the normal teenage years," she said in the matter-of-fact tone of someone who has devoted energy to analyzing and accepting her situation. Instead, she relied on her parents for emotional support and lived with them to protect her from the uncertainties of life with IBD.

"I wasn't able to go away to school," Marisa said. "My parents were the only ones who understood what I was going through. At 15, it was virtually impossible to have that relationship with anyone outside my family." She felt as if her life had slowed down from the rapid pace she'd engaged in before her illness when she was a competitive swimmer. She delayed graduating from college until 24, and she was still living with her parents at 26 because of her ulcerative colitis.

"As one psychiatrist that I saw put it, 'This illness has become like a permanent umbilical cord,'" she told me.

Ultimately, Marisa met a man with a son who had Crohn's disease, and they moved in together, finally ratifying her adulthood and readiness to enter the world outside the protection of her family home.

Because an invisible but powerful umbilical cord is formed as soon as the diagnosis comes down, criticism or blame from a parent to a child over IBD can be devastating. As I described earlier in the book, the ongoing conflict between my mother and me spilled over into the arena of my ulcerative colitis. When I went home to recover from a particularly bad flare, my mother let me know that it wouldn't be happening to me if I cared more about other people and less about myself. I internalized the message that the disease was a function of my inadequacy. I decided to enter therapy to deal with my deep connection to a critical mother, a thorny relationship that I was sure was exacerbating my colitis.

If your parents are overly anxious or even critical, as some parents become when they feel out of control and are desperate to regain it, you may appreciate their support. However, understand that it comes at a cost. Your sense of powerlessness over the disease is compounded by your lack of control over your own life. You can experience internal gridlock, which creates stress, and that can aggravate the symptoms.

"I hate their sympathy," said Diana, 30, a woman who was diagnosed with ulcerative colitis in high school. "I absolutely hate it." She knows how to handle her flares, and after a lengthy period of time, she usually improves. "In the meantime, I don't want them to ask me how I am. It's like a broken record. It makes me feel bad. 'Did you do take your medicine? Did you call the doctor?' It makes me feel 15 again."

Intense Parental Management

Mount Sinai's Dr. Reigada, a clinical psychologist who also teaches at Brooklyn College, sees many parents who are "over-protective and over-controlling." They take over the medical management of their children's IBD "during the adolescent years, when they're supposed to be separating, when adolescents should start managing themselves and their medications," she said. "It's not the best approach for anxious kids, and it fuels anxiety. Kids need to feel competent in their own ability to manage themselves and their own illness."

Carol and Gina's mother/daughter relationship was focused on who was in charge of Gina's Crohn's disease. Carol's anxieties over her daughter's illness virtually took over her own life and beleaguered her daughter's. Carol's fear mutated into certainty that her daughter never had Crohn's until she started taking medication for it.

"My mother analyzes me to death and is a huge part of the disease," Gina said. "She's been trying to fix me. Every time she talks to somebody, I end up going to another practitioner: acupuncture, herbalists, psychologists, different remedies, another herbalist. She does so much research. She used to take me to all my doctor's appointments. It changed her life more than it changed mine. She's still trying to fix me, but ever since I got my own car, I'd go to the doctor by myself. When I went to college, I started paying for doctors' appointments."

Gina expresses a mixture of self-interest and empathy for what her parents must be feeling, and self-awareness that she had to submit to the will of her anxious mother.

"There are times I wanted to get mad at her, but she was keeping me alive," Gina said. "I couldn't alienate her, so I could never have a huge blowup. I'd always hold my tongue more than I wanted to. I needed her to buy my meds, be with me, care for me. I'd apologize more than I wanted to. I know it was tough for her and my dad." Gina was able to declare her emotional autonomy, a testament both to her determination and to her mother's ultimate willingness to let go.

Gina exemplifies the divided feelings of children toward overwrought parents, something that is widespread in IBD parent/child relationships. Children's desire to take control of their own lives can be at odds with their needs and their desire to be taken care of. It takes a skillful parent and a secure adolescent or young adult to dance this dance of ambivalence.

The fear of becoming too dependent on your parents can diminish as you gradually gain an inner sense of security and individuality. You find outside sources of support so as not to be too reliant. Adina, away from home at college, depended on a local friend's mother rather than her own when she needed help during her flares. "I was off on my own, getting used to that, and it was hard to admit I needed help. You're just coming out of your teenage years and you don't want to go back to needing your mom." As she matured and developed a firmer sense of self, however, her feeling of being threatened for depending on her mother declined. "By the time I was in graduate school and had to come home when I had flares, I could then admit I needed more help."

Living away from home still doesn't guarantee that young adults with IBD will feel self-sufficient. Being pulled back into the childhood home when you get sick means the umbilical cord isn't completely severed. Nerissa, who was diagnosed with Crohn's at age 22, worked as a newspaper reporter, lived in her own place, and felt she was on the road to a fully adult life. While she appreciates her parents' support during her rough years with the disease, it clearly frustrates her that she needed them beyond the age when she thought she would.

Nerissa said she asked her parents to accompany her to doctors' appointments because she felt her memory was impaired — collateral damage from her severe Crohn's. "Half of me wanted to be independent and half of me was dependent on my parents to look after me," she said. At the same time, Nerissa likes knowing that her parents will take care of her if she needs them. "If anything goes wrong, and I needed to come back home, they'd be incredibly supportive."

Another facet of the child/parent dynamic occurs when your parents are frightened that if they lose control over you, your disease will get worse. "My parents were always scared," recalled Rachel. "The hardest part for my parents was when I was 16, still having regular flare-ups. But I wanted to start having boyfriends and going out. You try to become an adult a bit more. You are bit of a rebel. They worried a lot. If I started to do silly things, would that make me more ill?

"When I was 18 [the legal drinking age in England, where she lives], they worried that if I decided to drink, I'd basically be killing myself," she continued. "They also worried I would try to do too much and exhaust myself. And they wouldn't be able to stop it."

Positive Dynamics

As many troublesome relationships as there are, there are many positive ones as well. The balance between parental support and young-adult independence can work well when both child and parent demonstrate exceptionally strong and balanced temperaments. Benjamin, who was diagnosed with Crohn's at 16, and his mother, Sharon, have a relationship that strikes a balance between angst and, as he puts it, "not smothering. My mom knew when to leave me alone and was very supportive that I go out with my friends and do whatever I wanted. We had a very good dynamic. Those growing pains that kids might go through were never a big deal. I was just happy with my mom helping me out. She didn't bother me. She trusted me to tell her when things were going wrong."

Chelsea has good memories of the way her parents treated her when she became ill with Crohn's at 13. "I look back on it now and am so thankful for the way they dealt with it," she said. "They were obviously very worried about me. They'd take me to a shopping mall after I was in the hospital. Half the time, I wasn't well enough to be walking around. I never felt they were overdoing it so much that I'd feel like I wasn't normal. I was volunteering at Mount Sinai [Hospital] in the children's IBD unit. You see all kinds of parents, all kinds of parenting, the way people deal with it. Keeping a good head on your shoulders and not scaring your child is very important. Lots of times, I didn't know what was going on and my parents didn't either. They helped me stay calm and get through it all."

Josh, the 6-year-old whose Crohn's was so serious that he apologized to his mom for having to give him an enema, has grown up with the help of his mother, Jacque. "This past summer, I moved to the beach for three months," he said. "Not having her there, I realized she had already shown me everything I needed to do to take care of myself. I think she's really showed me how to be a Crohn's patient. She showed me the best way to eat, the way I should cook my food, how to take my medicine. She showed me that when I feel something going on, not to be afraid to call the doctor. I have all their phone numbers. If I needed to go to the hospital, I could go without her, and I have all my information with me. If I needed to move out now, I could and hold my own with my disease." Josh had a sense of calm and pride that he was taking over his own care at 22.

Not Telling Them

Nevertheless, even parents with the best intentions may inadvertently weaken their children's trust in them as confidantes and caretakers. Tiffany, who was diagnosed with Crohn's at 16, says her mother violated her privacy by discussing her IBD with a wide group of friends and acquaintances, thereby breaching her trust. Tiffany said she understands why her mother consulted others. "She needed information and they all had it," she said. But Tiffany resented going to synagogue and having a man she had never met before approach her to ask what dose of medication she was on. "Someone comes over to me and says, 'Oh, you've been on 60 milligrams of 6MP. How's that going for you?' I was like, 'Well, we haven't seen any results yet.' 'Well, I'm on 150, and it may take eight months before you feel better,' he said and he walked away. I had no idea who this person was."

Tiffany said that's when she cut her parents out of "the whole process. I rewrote my chart, saying they no longer had permission to talk to my doctor without my consent. They're my parents, and they want to know what goes on with me. If they ask me how I am, I say 'fine,' even if I'm having a flare, because I don't want to discuss minor problems with them."

When parents unwittingly shower their anxiety on you, one of the solutions is to deal with your condition yourself. "My mom has always not only harbored a lot guilt but desperately wanted to fix it," said Hannah, 24, a tiny, attractive woman who was diagnosed with Crohn's at 12. "My dad was the stable one, saying, 'Let's all calm down. You've gone through a lot.' She'd get really frustrated with my doctor and yell at him, 'She's still sick!' and my dad was the voice of reason." Hannah avoided triggering her mother's anxieties when she was in college by not telling her when she got sick, but the penalty she paid was not getting her mother's support. Her father had died suddenly years earlier and he was no longer around to calm things down.

Ben had his own way of keeping his mother from jumping into action when he didn't want her to. "I'm somewhat protective about how much I talk about with my mom, because if I tell her I'm having a rough day and don't feel well, she'll overreact," he said. He feels confident that he can manage his illness himself, he added. "I know whether it's very bad or something that will pass. She's a little more alarmist."

Conclusion

The term "Gordian knot" is used metaphorically to describe an extremely difficult or complex problem. It perfectly captures the situation between young adults with IBD and their parents. As a side note, I noticed as I researched this issue on the Internet that no matter how I entered the subject in the search engine, the results were almost always parent-centered, such as, how can parents cope with a chronically ill child or a child with IBD? I could find little or no material written to help children with IBD deal with family dynamics.

While many young people I interviewed had no difficulty with their parents and welcomed their support and expertise, others found their parents' attention smothering and intrusive. Their ambivalence toward needing care and rejecting it created problems well past their teens.

Nevertheless, as children age, perspectives change. Those who struggle with IBD and their parents seem to make their way through the difficult years of adolescence and young adulthood and find their way to reconciliation and peace. Those who have had no struggle seem happy and well adjusted, despite their disease. Everyone has good intentions. No one wants to be hurtful. The task for both children and parents in the tough times with IBD is how to communicate with calmness, patience and love.

CHAPTER ELEVEN

How Parents Cope

When one of my children told me that he'd had rectal bleeding for two months, I felt myself immediately gripped by acute anxiety. I had been at high alert because of my medical history, but now I flashed on a radically different future for this young adult ready to make his way in the world. If he had IBD, his plans would be put on hold, throwing us together to handle his medical needs when he was more than ready to separate from me. IBD would cast a pall over his life and mine.

As it turned out, a colonoscopy showed bleeding internal hemorrhoids. But even that brief brush with the possibility of having a child with IBD and all its implications gave me an insight into what parents of children with Crohn's disease and ulcerative colitis have to confront much of the time.

It is unimaginably difficult to witness IBD's physical and psychological assaults on your child. This would be true no matter what the chronic illness, but IBD is especially insidious, both socially and emotionally.

"When a child is diagnosed with IBD, the entire family is affected," wrote researchers in the Journal of Developmental Behavioral Pediatrics. They lay out the challenges, including the need to incorporate "multiple IBD medications, each with a different dosing schedule, into one's daily routine. [Parents] must also alter their schedules to accommodate frequent medical appointments and unexpected hospitalizations and surgeries."

The researchers go on to write that the unpredictable nature of IBD and its symptoms "may cause families to live in a constant state of uncertainty, never knowing when symptoms will... disrupt family functioning. Many [parents] also worry about the impact of IBD on their child's future, further increasing parenting stress." (Gray, 2014)

Impact of the Diagnosis

Upon your child's diagnosis with Crohn's or colitis, your challenges are immediate, and the impact on you is immense and wide-ranging. Some parents are so shaken by the diagnosis that they describe a feeling of unreality. One mother related that at the beginning, she waited to be awakened from a nightmare. (Hordvik, 1998) Other parents immediately snap into action and become deeply involved in every aspect of the disease. "Am I an obsessed mother or what?" Carol asked rhetorically about her preoccupation with her daughter's Crohn's disease.

Just as there are said to be stages of grieving, parents go through a similar process after learning that their child has IBD. The first emotion is usually relief that the symptoms finally have a name. Then, almost immediately, a deep anguish emerges, alternating with grit, determination, and dread. "I went through stages of acceptance, being in shock, in survival mode," said Amy after her son, Jesse, was diagnosed with ulcerative colitis at age 6. "I was depressed about it, not clinically, but in the doldrums, being angry and sad. On my drive to work, I'd burst into tears. My childhood was easy. I never had to worry about this stuff. It'll never be that way for him."

Sometimes, after the diagnosis, parents acquire new insight into their child's reaction to their illness. Mary had been unaware of the trepidation her 11-year-old daughter, Katherine, felt after hearing that she had Crohn's. Then she saw Katherine's shoulders relax and saw her exhale in relief when the doctor sat her down and said, "This will not kill you."

"I hadn't realized up to that point just how worried she'd been," Mary said. "That broke my heart. I had been trying hard to help her, but I didn't understand how scared she was."

Another mother discovered her 15-year-old son's strength of character by watching the way he handled his newly diagnosed Crohn's disease. Denise had posted a photograph on Facebook of her son, Jordan, wearing a feeding tube and, triumphantly if wearily, holding up a football trophy. He had already been quickly transformed from a healthy high school football player to a thin-as-a-rail boy who couldn't hold down his food.

"I'm a basket case," she said. "We're literally worn out. I can't help him and how excruciating that is. All I can do is reassure him that we'll get him back to a state where he's a little bit healthier." When Jordan returned to his Alabama high school with the feeding tube, a girl said to him, "I feel so sorry for you," Denise related. Jordan looked at the girl and said, "Don't feel sorry for me. You can pray for me. I'm all right. I'm going to be okay." "That makes me cry as a mother," Denise said. "He's that good of a man, to handle this and not let the disease become him."

Gathering Information and Making Decisions

After the diagnosis of IBD, one of the first decisions a parent has to make is whether to accumulate extensive information about the disease or to try to avoid being overwhelmed by the contradictory assertions on the Internet about the best way to treat the disease. "There are people who do well with lots of information," said Cathy, a therapist and the mother of a son with Crohn's disease. "Some people want to know every little thing that could happen. Other people, the more you tell them, the more anxious they get. I'm in that second group."

However, Jeffrey, a single father, wanted to learn everything he could about his daughter Maggie's Crohn's disease. Immediately upon receiving the diagnosis, he disregarded the doctor's advice to stay away from the Internet. He compiled a huge dossier on the disease. Some of it was helpful to him, but some left him feeling angry and helpless after doctors rejected the nontraditional treatments he'd found online. "It was like a body blow," he said of Maggie's diagnosis and the aftermath. Because of his research, he said, he "knew it was a life-changing thing for both of us. I knew what it meant and what the future was going to hold for us." The hard-case scenarios he'd read about turned out to apply to his daughter. "Unfortunately, she's a rather severe case," he said. "She's been in the hospital a number of times and has an ileostomy."

Although it would seem that more research would bring more insight, parental research does have its limits. There are so many problems that resist online solutions and parents confront these issues almost every day. For example, if your child is old enough to take on self-care, how involved should you be with his or her illness? How do you know whether your child is complying with the pills, enemas, infusions, and injections and whatever else the doctor has prescribed? What if your child is noncompliant? How much of an inspector can you afford to be without driving your child away? If your relationship is generally positive, how can you best support your sick child, keep your child's spirits up and not let despair take over? How can you shield your child from your own fear about the long-term effects of medication and the ravaging effect of these autoimmune diseases on your child's body?

If only there were a manual that provided answers. With little or no prior experience dealing with an unstable condition, parents try to apply intuition, compassion, and tough love when appropriate and then hope that they've taken the right approach. And, above all, they try to contain themselves when the disease gives them every reason to express their stress and anxiety.

Responding to IBD

Simone Leo, a social worker with Crohn's disease and ulcerative colitis, volunteered at the CCFA's Camp Oasis for children with IBD in Elizaville, N.Y. At camp, she witnessed what happens when parents don't contain their anxiety. "There was a child who was really upset and didn't think she could make it here," Leo recalled as she sat in the camp's social hall. "When her parents dropped her off, they were crying hysterically. Children learn from their parents' reactions. When the parents have high anxiety, the children do, too. The parents can cry," she added, "just not in front of their child."

Worrying about how your child will handle IBD away from you may seem perfectly logical. Being separated from your child may feel risky and dangerous. Your protective instinct kicks in. For example, some parents don't let their children sleep at friends' houses overnight for fear that they will have an accident or will forget to take their medications.

If the situation were less serious, parents might let their child experience the repercussions of forgetting necessary care. But with IBD, the stakes are high and the temptation for parents to exert control is difficult to resist. Once a flare happens, it's hard to make it go away. So parents are caught in a bind. If your child regularly forgets to take medication, it can put him or her into a spiral of decline. If your child tries to do too much or tries to appear too normal, the disease can get out of control.

Mental health professionals agree that how you handle IBD from the diagnosis onward and how you cope with your own massive lack of control over IBD's capricious ups and downs will have a significant impact on your child. "When some people get anxious, they become hyper-anxious," said Linda Sofer, a clinical social worker. "If you're constantly checking on your child, asking, 'Are you okay? Did you go to the bathroom? How many times?' Constantly asking or checking can foster too much dependence."

When Linda's son, Gideon, was 12, he underwent major abdominal surgery. "He recuperated and was feeling better and, two months later, there was a school ski trip," she recalled. "He wanted to go. My first reaction was, 'You can't go.' I spoke with his doctor, who said, 'Look, of course he'll be at higher risk than a child who's completely healthy, but he's well enough to be on this ski trip.'" Her son was determined that his illness would not stop him from doing things. "He had a great time," Linda said. "He became a downhill skier.'"

In another case, Mary knew that her young daughter, Kathleen, did not want to take responsibility for her Crohn's disease. "It was up to me to get her to take her meds," said Mary, who worked hard to keep Kathleen away from the surgeon's knife. "I would have let her be on her own more if it wasn't so potentially damaging." Now that

Kathleen is in her 20s, her mother is more relaxed. "She's totally on it, very involved with her doctors and managing well," Mary said. "I couldn't do any better than what she's doing for herself."

Aside from your worries, you may also bear persistent feelings of guilt. Fran, for example, harbored fear that in trying to heal her daughter, she might have allowed her to be harmed in the long run. "I have to live with the guilt that they put toxins in her body for a long time," Fran said, looking into an uncertain future and feeling unsettled about what she saw. "I feel terrible. I'm worried she'll have a baby with no arms. I hope to God that isn't true, but I carry that."

The mother of an 11-year-old with ulcerative colitis told researchers, "You blame yourself. What did you do that gave your child this problem? The answer is nothing. But you feel guilty. As a parent you feel it's your job to keep your child safe and well and you can't, because you have no control over the disease." Her prescription for parents is to talk about it. "You are not alone. Never bottle it up." (Hordvik, 1998) As true as this advice is for young people with IBD, it is just as valid for their parents.

You can help forge your child's character by reacting to each twist of IBD with calmness, something I struggled with internally when I had that IBD scare with my son. You can positively influence the quality of your relationship with your child as well as your child's emotional stability. How you respond will also affect you as parents and individuals. Your challenge is to balance your child's considerable needs with your desire to attend to your own needs and those of your spouse and other children.

"When a child is given this kind of diagnosis, the parents should consult a mental health professional as part of the workup," said Dr. Robert Kravis, a pediatric psychologist who practices in Elkins Park, Pennsylvania and has children with disabilities in his practice. "They may not actually need or want therapy, but it's crucial that they be connected so they can use the professional if the need arises. The strain that this kind of thing puts on the parental relationship and family is not easy to sort out if there are other children as well. There is no formula."

Many parents take a thoughtful approach to interacting with their child with IBD and they find it helpful to have underlying principles and values that work best for the child.

Jacque took a position akin to tough love. "Crohn's was never an allowable excuse not to do homework, not to live life," she said, referring to her son Josh. "I don't have the 'I feel sorry for you' gene. I am a very cuddly, compassionate person, but if I felt sorry for him instead of helping him, he wouldn't be the person he is today."

Naomi and David also decided early on that they would not coddle their son, Elijah. "We decided that Elijah was a kid who happened to have Crohn's, but it wasn't going to dictate his life," Naomi said. "I didn't want to become a *chalaria,*" she added, referring to the Yiddish term for a nervous, anxious person. She noted the presence of hypochondriacs in the family, "and," she said, "It was our job to help Elijah learn how to cope with it and have as normal a life as possible." One arena in which Naomi and David drew boundaries was around school. They judged Elijah's capacity to handle school by pure instinct. They had to assess when to tell Elijah he had to go to school even for a few hours when he complained about stomach pain and when to relent and allow him to languish on the couch.

There is so much static in interactions between parents and healthy children that it is hard to know, with kids who have IBD, when the disease or medication (particularly Prednisone) is the cause of the friction and when the conflict just reflects the healthy process of individuation.

In order to encourage independence, which also applies to being the parent of a healthy teenager and young adult, the ideal approach is to be helpful without being intrusive. How baffling it can be to decide when to refrain from intervening and when to intercede from a place of concern and love, not from anxiety and fear.

Dr. Kravis observes that parents and their sick children may fall into arguing about some task going undone when the real issue is that the child is having a hard time accepting IBD and its impact. "I think people would rather fight about something they can influence than something they can't," he said. "Sometimes, this is a kid's way of saying, 'I can control what I do and don't do' when they feel out of control with their bowels. If the parents could see that, then maybe they'd handle that issue differently and talk about the feeling of wanting to be in control rather than whether the kid is going to do their homework or not."

Setting Boundaries

Some parents talked about their internal struggle to maintain healthy boundaries while fervently wishing at the same time that they could intervene. Rosa, whose son Ben, now 30, was diagnosed with Crohn's during his junior year of college, said that her immediate instinct was to sweep in, take over, and find an answer. "You look at your kid and you think, he's got this life sentence," she said. "[When he was first diagnosed,] a part of me felt invincible, proactive, motherly." Now, she acknowledges that his Crohn's "teaches me to act differently than is my normal inclination, which is to think I have the answer to everything." She said she urgently wants to tell him, 'You should eat better and take probiotics and see an acupuncturist and go to the doctor, for God's sake. You should take Pilates and yoga classes.'" She paused and added a little sadly, "Those are not my decisions."

Ben's parents would seem to fit a certain stereotype of the involved mother and the more detached father. Ben described his father, Fred, as being more interested in getting something to eat and watching a football game than in involving himself in his son's Crohn's disease. Fred explained himself: "The more anxiety that Rosa communicated, the less I communicated. Of course I was concerned, although I didn't have tremendous anxiety. I felt he was under a doctor's care. He was responding and he was going to be fine. That's what I told myself and that's how I felt."

Liz expressed the frustration of many parents regarding the impasse they confront with college-age children. "I was trying to make it better for Andrew by taking over the management and the stress," she said. Then, she added, she realized: "It's his disease. But I'd be doing the reading and research. I want him to step forward and learn about it." She said she hopes he will be "mature enough and smart enough to reach out and figure these things on his own. He's 23. He's got to take it on."

Finding a Way out of Dependence

Understandably, many parents hope that over time, their maturing child will assume responsibility for decisions about medical treatment, eating, drinking alcohol, stress levels, and other ancillary issues related to IBD. (You can make your own wish list.) They take stock of their child's capacity for self-care and recognize their child's need for independence. Of course, this is more easily accomplished when the disease is mild or in remission. Still, short of dire illness, most parents feel ready to shed their authority role and let the young adult take over. Potential problems arise, however, when a child is unwilling or unable to handle the tasks necessary to control the disease. Then IBD can breed dependency on parents for far longer than would be the case if the child were healthier. Love, caretaking, and kinship can easily evolve into an unhealthy attachment.

The long-term commitment that parents make to children with IBD can create battle fatigue for both parent and child. Parents are afraid for their children and they may cling to their children, just as their children cling to them. After a while, one party is ready to disengage. And it's not always the child.

Sharon, who has managed her own Crohn's disease for decades, feels somewhat impatient when her daughter, Hannah, who also has Crohn's, regularly calls her mother at 5:30 a.m. to ask what she should eat that day. "She's 23," Sharon said, clearly feeling encumbered. "She feels at a loss. She wakes up and knows she has to go to work. She's nauseous, but if she doesn't eat, she'll be too lightheaded to function. But why is she asking me what to eat? She has to feel powerful enough to be independent. But that's cut short completely when she's not feeling well."

When Linda's son, Gideon, asked her to wash some of the components of his feeding tube, she was about to comply but then she stopped. "He is suffering but also getting pulled into this dependence on me," she recalled. Fostering independence is one of the biggest challenges of parenting a totally healthy child. When children are sick with IBD, parents become torn between their instinct to help and comfort their children and their understanding of the importance of helping their children to become better at taking care of themselves.

Fearing that her son, Joseph, could die because he was neglecting his serious Crohn's disease, Karen nevertheless got angry with him when he called her at work complaining that his stomach hurt. She knew he hadn't taken his medicine. It wasn't for her lack of effort. She put his medicine in a weekly container and wrote down the schedule when he had to take it. "I start work at 7 a.m. and I'd call him and say, 'Did you take your medicine?' Inside, I'd feel angry that he's 16 and capable of taking care of himself. Why do I have to do this?" she would ask herself. Then she would feel guilty for her anger.

Like many parents and kids with IBD, Fran, a psychologist, and her daughter Hannah got caught "in a complicated place with her emotions and my emotions," Fran recalled. "Hannah needed to be going through separation and individuation, but she was sick and in need of my help. In the morning, we'd be in the bathroom when she was in pain and I'd be late to work. I'd have to cancel patients to take her to the doctor. Her emotions were raw, as were mine." Fran's husband had died suddenly, just before Hannah was diagnosed. Fran added, "She'd call me when she needed me, and she needed me a lot, more than she wanted and more than I wanted her to need me."

One day, their tensions came to a head. After one too many phone calls from Hannah, Fran answered the phone with, "Now what?" Hannah wouldn't talk to her for two weeks, saying, with adolescent hyperbole, that it was the cruelest thing her mother had ever said to her.

Fran was too weary to argue. "There just wasn't that much I could do," she said years later. "I was pretty depleted. There were times she obviously needed something from me, but couldn't take in anything I had to offer." Hannah told her mother that she didn't need her to do anything. She just wanted Fran to be empathetic and a good listener. They reconciled, of course, but the worry about her daughter's health never stops for Fran.

Sharon, whose 23-year-old daughter, Hannah, calls her frequently, tries to be supportive but she also recognizes the fine line between being helpful and being too interconnected. She watched a video about the difference between empathy and sympathy and took in the message. "Empathy feels a person's pain," she said. "Sympathy feels as if you're separate. If you're too empathetic, you can go down with your child."

Fran, as a psychologist, also understands the difference between sympathy and empathy. "We want our children to be healthy. We want to fix them and protect them," she said. "One of the hardest things for parents with a child with a disease like this is that there's practically nothing you can do short of love them and support them."

Making Sacrifices

Parents will indeed go to great lengths to try to fix their child's condition. Some will even sacrifice their own comfort and wellbeing to provide for their child. Martha, for example, practiced sticking a needle into her own thigh before giving injections of growth hormone to her daughter, Emily, whose Crohn's disease had caused her to stop growing. "I couldn't bring myself to do that," said her husband, Albert. "Our daughter was very appreciative of her courage." Martha's reasoning was matter of fact. "It was such a crisis for us. It's like being in a bunker. You're just focused on her survival. I really wasn't aware of a lot of stuff beyond the physical and doing what the doctor said to get her well."

Unfortunately, some parents metaphorically or literally don't nourish themselves while throwing themselves into their child's care, thus jeopardizing their own health. The morning after her 12-year-old son, Jeffrey, had a feeding tube inserted into his stomach to heal his virulent Crohn's disease, Heathir collapsed on his bed from anemia, dehydration, and malnourishment. "I only had so much money for food," Heathir recalled later, after her economic situation had improved. "Jeffrey would get first choice of food, Annie (his sister, who also developed Crohn's) second and all that was left was rice and that's what I was eating. I was going without." Jeffrey stayed in the hospital until his mother, who had been admitted to the room next to his, was discharged. This could be viewed as either as noble self-sacrifice or not taking seriously enough the need to maintain one's strength so as to function as the parent and caretaker.

Dr. Kravis observed that many parents suffer "an enormous injury to think they're produced a defective child. The parents feel responsible, particularly the mother who gave birth to such a child. She has to atone or make amends or sacrifices because she's responsible. I'm not talking about the reality" of the situation, he said. The mother unconsciously feels that "this child came from me and is damaged."

When parents feel terrible for leaving their child alone in the hospital, they have to step up and be the grownups, said Dr. Kodman-Jones. "As adults, we're supposed to be able to tolerate that guilt," she said. "We're the adults. We need to hold it together. To say that if I stay in the hospital,

I'll feel less guilty," is the wrong approach, she said. Left alone, "the teen will talk with the nurses. They'll build a little psychological muscle dealing with hospital staff and become more independent and be more in charge of their illness."

Handling themselves away from parents also has an impact on how young people with IBD manage their pain, she said. She described seeing "kids in a flare, in pain and cramping. The kids are telling their parents how much pain they're in. The parent leaves. The kid gets on the phone with a friend and it doesn't look like they're in pain. Are they making it up? No. When left to their own devices, they'll talk to their friends to help themselves and handle their pain."

Stress on Marriage

When so much worry and attention by one parent is focused on the child with IBD, marriages can suffer. Often, the other parent feels neglected or there is disagreement about how to handle the sick child. "One parent coddles. The other lays down the law. That creates tension between the two parents," said Dr. Kravis.

This is particularly true when one is not the biological parent of the sick child. "It's very difficult on my second marriage," said Laura. "It's been horrible for my husband. He feels like I'm enabling Thomas. He feels as though Thomas comes first, then my job and somewhere he and our daughter fit in. I think he feels deprived and that I deprive our daughter. But Thomas does come first. I think that's a common feeling in families, that the squeaky wheel gets all the grease."

Dr. Kravis notes that mothers in a second marriage may try to compensate the child for "the lousy things that have happened to him or her. This can build up a great deal of resentment in the new spouse. This is another reason why it's really important for people to be connected with mental health services. The illness turns up the heat tremendously."

Conclusion

Below are some suggestions about how to promote your maturing child's independence and self-reliance and how to take care of yourself at the same time.

- Include the child in all the information meetings and information sharing by doctors and the health-care team and prepare them to be part of the discussions.
- Don't keep secrets about the health-care situation of the teenager.
- Plan to give the child time alone with the doctor; one possibility, if there's enough time, is to structure time alone for the doctor and the young person, then for the doctor and the parents, and then all together.
- Give young people time to think about decisions that need to be made.
- If children want to talk about their IBD with a sibling or friend, don't stand in their way.
- If an argument starts, suggest trying a different approach, like writing down the pros and cons, asking a third person to join you, writing a note to each other, or cooling off for a few minutes and then trying again, a strategy developed by psychologist Donald Brunnquell, director of the Office of Ethics for Children's Hospitals and Clinics of Minnesota.

- Seek professional mental health counseling when you feel that you're at an impasse with your child or your spouse as a result of tension over IBD. "Parents should not think of counseling as addressing a dysfunction," said Linda Sofer, a licensed clinical social worker. "It's a way to get families communicating and understanding each other if they're having difficulty."
- Put yourself on time-out when you feel you're about to lose your temper with your child. Even five minutes alone to regroup and breathe deeply can spare you from feeling guilty later, and you will spare your child from the stress of an angry confrontation.
- Expect the unexpected. If and when your child's IBD suddenly acts up, maintain your calm. You've gotten through hard times before and you'll get through this one. Becoming agitated will not help you or your child.
- Reach out. Talk about your anxiety with friends. Open up and vent your stress. Find a group sponsored by the Crohn's & Colitis Foundation of America (CCFA). Attend meetings to learn about others' experiences with IBD, to talk about yours, or just to listen.
- Take care of yourself physically and emotionally. Someone else needs you, not just your child with IBD, but also your spouse, if you have one, your other children, and your friends. Make it a priority to take time for you and them.
- Determine what activities are realistic for your child to master. Your child may feel inadequate and incapable because of the limitations imposed by IBD. If

you're having trouble making that assessment, seek medical or mental health counseling.

"You just do the best you can," Sharon said, adding that she was resigned to the enigma of dealing with her daughter's stress over IBD. "Kids aren't perfect. Parents aren't perfect. Even if we parents mess up sometimes, kids just need to feel that we're trying."

CHAPTER TWELVE
Surgery

It was a beautiful spring day when I took a call from my gastroenterologist. He was brusque and to the point. My colonoscopies had shown dysplasia, precancerous cells, in the same location for three years in a row. I would need to have my entire colon removed as soon as possible to prevent colon cancer. He didn't linger on the phone. He was clearly uncomfortable delivering the news. I hung up in shock, devastated.

Why was this happening? I'd controlled my symptoms for almost a decade and I thought I was okay. I'd lived with ulcerative colitis for 33 years. This was the latest sucker punch to be delivered by my disease. And yet, it wasn't a total surprise. I had long feared this moment. A total colectomy, the removal of my entire colon, and a colostomy bag were the specters I'd dreaded since my mother guaranteed they would be my fate if I continued to eat (insert name of any food I liked). It had finally happened.

I cried, wiped away my tears, and faced my new reality. I began to do research. I learned that a colostomy bag was no longer my only option. I could have an internal pouch, called a J-pouch, fashioned from the end of my small intestine that would function like a mini-colon. It would enable me to use the toilet, although my stool would be liquid and I would assume the risk of pouchitis, an inflammation of the pouch. I didn't care. I found a surgeon who had done many J-pouch surgeries in Philadelphia. The night before my colon was removed, friends gathered at my home and offered blessings to carry me into surgery. I felt supported and loved, and the ritual helped me through an uncertain and scary time.

In the recovery area, my surgeon told me that my entire colon looked like a battlefield. I asked to see my colon, now out of my body, to see the organ that had harassed me since childhood. He said it was impossible. So, I never got to say goodbye and good riddance. And I never thanked my colon, face to face, for helping to make me the person I had become.

The next three months before the second surgery were miserable. I wore a temporary colostomy bag that leaked and bedeviled me and my boyfriend, soon-to-be my husband. I counted the days until the bag would be gone.

During the second surgery, the surgeon attached the end of my small intestine to my rectal muscles, which enabled food to travel quickly through me after being absorbed by the small intestine. Afterward, I needed to go to the emergency room twice — once for a bowel obstruction soon after the second surgery and a second time because I carelessly ate popcorn and gave myself another bowel obstruction. Since then, I've learned to eat slowly, to chew my food thoroughly and to be careful not to exert myself within an hour or so after eating to prevent nausea. Otherwise, I've had no complications. My husband and I toast my surgeon on every anniversary of my surgery. I am grateful to be alive.

My story is by no means universal. Most patients I spoke with who underwent surgery had had runaway symptoms that were resistant to multiple medications before they were told that surgery was the only alternative. Following surgery, many Crohn's patients continue to take medication and many with ulcerative colitis suffer from pouchitis, which they treat with antibiotics and anti-inflammatory medication, while those with ostomies feel immensely relieved to bid goodbye to their IBD symptoms.

When surgery loomed, I actually felt fortunate that I had ulcerative colitis. Although removing a major organ is an extreme panacea, it was possible because ulcerative colitis is located only in the large intestine and does not spread anywhere else.

With Crohn's disease, however, surgery is a stopgap measure, not the potential end of the disease. Crohn's can spread anywhere from the mouth to the anus, although it is often located in the small intestine, which absorbs nutrients and is not expendable. So resection, or partial surgery, is the way — at least, temporarily — to resolve intractable inflammation. Surgeons may cut away pieces of diseased small intestines many times over a patient's lifetime. And there is quite a bit of small bowel to cut away. In an adult male, the small bowel is more than 22 feet long; in an adult female, it is more than 23 feet long and, in children, it is 18 to 20 feet long.

According to the CCFA, up to 45 percent of people with ulcerative colitis will eventually require surgery, and up to 75 percent of people with Crohn's disease will also require surgery. Crohn's patients who undergo one surgery are likely to need another in 10 to 15 years.

Let's define the surgical terms. An ileostomy is the opening created by the surgeon to bring the small intestine (ileum) to the surface of the abdomen. This may be temporary or permanent. A colostomy is the opening created by the surgeon to bring the colon (large intestine) to the surface of the abdomen. In both cases, stool drains into a removable, disposable bag called a colostomy or ileostomy bag, which is held flush against your body to permit the sanitary collection and disposal of bodily wastes. Since the output contains digestive enzymes, it can be highly irritating if stool gets on the skin. Barriers that sit flush against the skin are designed to protect the skin from coming into contact with the output.

With the end of your intestine protruding from your abdomen and draining into an ostomy bag, you are actually looking at the lining of your intestine, which looks a lot like the inside of your cheek. This up-close-and-personal look at my intestine unhinged me when I wore the bag.

Sometimes, an ostomy can be reversed, in cases where the doctor is using it to let your intestine rest for a few months. You use the bag while you recover from surgery. Then you may have another surgery to reattach the ends of the intestine so you no longer need the ostomy. This is called a reversal. Sometimes, an ileostomy is done as the first step in forming an ileal-anal reservoir, the J-pouch.

Maureen, who was diagnosed with ulcerative colitis at 15 and who had her colon removed at age 22, had to make a decision about whether to keep her ostomy or undergo a second surgery to get a J-pouch. She recounted what it was like to be "faced at a young age with having an ostomy. I don't know anybody who doesn't try to have an alternative. Once I had the ostomy, I hated having it. But I loved not being sick.

"In between surgeries, I postponed the reversal for a month because I felt so much better," she continued. Like many others who had read horror stories on the Internet about pouchitis, Maureen was worried about potential complications from a J- pouch. "It was a completely emotional reaction. I was panicked that I'd go back to the way it was. The surgeon made me realize that this wasn't going to happen, that [the second surgery] was the easy part and I'd feel better."

After her surgeries, Maureen had an epiphany. "I didn't realize how sick I had been until I felt better," she said. "Oh my God, this is what healthy people feel like? I didn't even remember. Wow! Who knew?" Still, she said, she understands why others might decide to quit after the first surgery and choose the ostomy over a J-pouch. She's just glad she didn't.

Colin was also nervous before he had a total colectomy to rid himself of his debilitating ulcerative colitis. The sight of his surgeon didn't boost his confidence. "I noticed he was wearing a button-down shirt, and he had buttoned his shirt wrong," Colin said with a dry laugh. "One of the last thoughts I had before I passed out was, 'He can't button his shirt right and he's going to perform an intricate removal of my colon?'"

After putting his life into the hands of a virtual stranger, Colin was not disappointed. "It's been great. Whenever someone asks me about my J-pouch, I say, 'This is how I have to live for the rest of my life, and I'll be perfectly happy. I'm not the same person I was when I was sick. I don't take any medication. I can control my bowel movements. It's a lot better than I was when sick."

Ostomies

Many patients are so grateful to have more control over their evacuation that they are happy to wear an ostomy bag. David reconsidered his initial decision to undergo two surgeries for a J-pouch. "The ostomy nurse was my age and she had an ostomy herself. I got great advice from her. The system I use now is the reason I decided to keep the ostomy. I have no issues with it. No issues with leakage. It doesn't bulge with gas or air, but it does become an issue when you dress a certain way. It does bother me, but I only kept it because I don't want the complications from the J pouch."

Surgery and its aftermath undoubtedly create physical trauma, but there are also emotional and social repercussions. For one thing, if you have a stoma, an opening in the abdomen for drainage purposes, you have to be trained to change the bag and to deal with leaks if they occur. If you are in a relationship, you may have to contend with a romantic partner who is less than enamored with the bag.

"Her bag was very difficult for me," said Hugo, whose wife had had surgery to rid her of rampant ulcerative colitis and who was waiting for a J- pouch. "I had a horrible time with that. I was not able to deal with it. You don't expect to see someone you love and live with have to go through that kind of procedure. I am a guy." In other words, a leaking ostomy bag is a turnoff.

At 25, Rachel had recently undergone surgery to cut out part of her small intestine, and she was wearing two ostomy bags. "The wound is opened up and the colon is spitting out bits of mucus. I empty the bag constantly. I'm so scared of it leaking," she said. Despite the unsavory aspects of her ostomy, she said, "I don't want to rely on going to the toilet anymore. I wish I'd known the surgery would make me feel this much better. I would have had it done years ago, but I was too frightened to have it done." She added that she is finished with having surgery for the time being and she is grateful to live with her ostomy.

Talking — or Not Talking — about the Bag or J-pouch

The upside to undergoing surgery is the control, either permanent or temporary, that you feel over your elimination system after years spent running to the bathroom and having no control over your bowels. Nevertheless, many people keep as a deep, dark secret the fact that they are wearing a bag to cover an abdominal opening that their intestines protrude through.

"It's almost easier to talk about cancer," said Michelle. "Nobody wants to hear about GI problems. If the subject ever comes up, I say, 'I don't have a colon. What don't you have?' You have to explain you have a pouch that's attached to your anus. I don't want to have that conversation. Skip it. But it is a part of everything you do. It's who you are."

On the other hand, reticence is not Maggie's style. She underwent surgery during her junior year of high school and transformed herself into a poster child for ostomates, as they are called. She has not only adjusted, she is dauntless about showing off her bag, and determined to do her small part to eradicate shame.

Maggie just wouldn't stay down after her surgery. Wearing a special belt, she was able to play soccer and swim while wearing the bag. Then, one day, not knowing anyone else with an ostomy, she took a camera "and decided to introduce myself on YouTube and Facebook. I just wanted to tell somebody." Her father, Jeffrey, has watched her with amazement. "She gets out a bullhorn and goes on the Internet. She's probably the most famous ostomy person in the world," he said, proudly. On one occasion, Maggie posed in a bikini and lifted her shirt, proudly showing off her bag.

Maggie also stands up to hints of harassment. Her father, Jeffrey, recounted a story Maggie had told him about walking down a hallway in college with her ostomy bag hanging out of the top of her pants. "This girl said to her, 'What's that thing?'" Jeffrey said. "She gave Maggie a lot of grief. 'Let me tell you what an ileostomy is for,'

Maggie replied. The girl was stunned. Maggie doesn't make any bones about it."

Clinton, who had also suffered with Crohn's disease, reached the summit of Mount Kiliminjaro while wearing an ostomy bag. He made the climb with other ostomates led by Rob Hill, who runs expeditions he calls "No Guts, Know Glory" to prove that young people with ostomies can accomplish anything they set their minds to.

When we spoke, Clinton described every nuance of the climb: the switchbacks, the steepness, the incredible beauty of the sunrise near the summit as well as his throwing up in thin air. He told me how taking Humira had put him into remission, which continues to the present time.

I waited. He hadn't mentioned his ostomy. I began to question whether he had one. Then I asked him about it. He hesitated, and then he replied haltingly, gathering steam as he talked. "I do have an ostomy. I did get surgery after a two-month hospital stay. I wasn't going to say anything about it. The girls I've been with know about it. A few of my friends know. I'm definitely not ashamed of it. It's kind of weird for me. It was supposed to be a temporary thing and now it's looking like it'll be a permanent thing. It hasn't stopped me from achieving anything and it's given me part of my health back. It's an important thing for people to know about it. I've spoken to huge auditoriums of people and said I have an ostomy.

"I didn't mean to sound like I was hiding it in any way," he went on, apologetically. "I just wasn't sure if I wanted to include it. But upon further speaking with you, I don't see a problem with that information being included in the book. I think it is a very important part of my story and it should be shared with others."

Clinton's painful ambivalence is striking and poignant. Being comfortable and unabashed about having your intestine literally exposed can be a huge undertaking, more formidable than climbing the highest mountain in Africa. After all, Clinton began wearing his ostomy bag at age 16, the age when boys approach sexual, if not emotional, maturity, and when fitting in and romance are everything.

Clinton said he had been "on death's door" before surgery. "When you're in it, you're not sure that's the case. People don't think you can die from Crohn's. They don't realize how serious it can get."

After Clinton initially had his ostomy surgery in January 2008, he recovered and was back at school "like nothing had happened," he said. "But of course I felt very alone since I didn't tell any of my friends. I was happy to be healthy and out of the hospital, but I still felt alone when dealing with something that no one really understood."

Marisa, another young person with IBD, is also reticent about her ostomy. "I would not tell anyone about the bag unless they had IBD or were close family members," she said. "I made sure my parents did not let on that I had a bag to any of their friends, so the whole hiding phase was extremely exhausting."

Jill, 25, has devoted her academic life to the study of young people with IBD. She was diagnosed with Crohn's disease at age 7 and she has undergone two surgeries since then. She is resigned about her own future. "I'm going to have a lot of surgery," she said. "Unfortunately, it's just about the right time that I have a third surgery. They say surgery gives you eight to 10 years until a relapse. I live a stressful lifestyle and have a social life, and if you said I need surgery now, I'd say I don't have the time. I'd need to wait until the summer. I need to wait until I'm financially stable before I can do it, and it's just the way it is. I know it's going to happen. You're just prepared for it."

Jill is also philosophical about her future. "I'll probably have colon cancer when I'm older. It's good that I know, because I'm prepared, almost. I have the attitude, 'Let's deal with it.' That's one of the questions I ask the kids I do research with: 'How does it feel having a disease that just won't go away? How do you feel about health problems in the future?'"

Living with Surgery

Not all IBD surgery involves cutting the colon. Some surgeries involve the insertion of feeding tubes, so young people can be fed a liquid diet directly into the stomach and they don't have to walk around in the school corridors with a nasogastric (NG) tube sticking out of their nose. Isabelle felt classmates staring at her in high school when she walked around with the NG tube, but with the gastric feeding tube, she said, "It's a tiny opening. You can't even see it if I wear a tight shirt, it's so tiny."

Surgery has become more refined in recent years, leaving fewer outward scars on the human body. Many patients now undergo laparoscopic surgery to remove their entire colon, leaving tiny incisions of 5 to 10 millimeters that can barely be seen post-surgery. Hannah has 15 incisions, all less than half an inch long and hardly visible. Adam also had laparoscopic surgery. "It wasn't pleasant but there's very little physical mark of it and not too much pain associated with it," he said. "I was in the hospital for five days. I try not to let Crohn's be a major factor in my life and I've been fortunate to deal with it, through sheer luck."

Facing Mortality

Mortality due to IBD is a sensitive subject. Some young people feel so ill that they worry about dying, and the fact that some people actually do die from the complications of Crohn's disease and ulcerative colitis is too frightening for their parents to contemplate. You rarely see an obituary attributing the death directly to Crohn's disease or ulcerative colitis, and the mortality rates for IBD are murky. According to Danish researcher Ebbe Langholz, the majority of the studies are limited by the fact that they looked at patients who were diagnosed and treated before the introduction of effective medications for IBD. (Langholz, 2010)

However, the most recent review of mortality studies related to IBD shows that the prognosis of Crohn's disease has not really changed in terms of mortality over the past 40 years, despite the introduction of more sophisticated medications. Researchers are waiting to see if the introduction of biologic medications will lead to a decrease in mortality or whether they will create an increase in the risk of mortality from the suppression of the immune system, which puts the body at risk of contracting other illnesses." (Langholz, 2010) The important thing to remember is that most people with IBD live a normal life span and continue to be treated with medication and surgery.

The mortality risk associated with ulcerative colitis derives mostly from the risk of colon cancer. But with annual colonoscopies and the close supervision of a physician, the cancer can be caught before it develops.

Gideon is a young man who died of a complication from Crohn's disease. He was an outlier among Crohn's patients in terms of the severity of his symptoms and — there is no way to get around it — his imprudent approach to caring for himself. Nevertheless, his struggles and aspirations are instructive.

After a severe recurrence of Crohn's symptoms required a six-month hospital stay and surgery during his senior year of high school, Gideon wore an ostomy bag for a time. He "was traumatized," his mother, Linda, said. "It was the most invasive thing physically for him."

By the time he was in college, a few years later, the ostomy had been reversed, but his symptoms remained severe. Gideon became determined to qualify for an intestinal transplant, a procedure very rarely performed and only considered for the sickest of sick patients. Living alone in California, across the country from his family, Gideon developed a fistula, but he refused to go to the hospital.

"He had this opening in his abdomen," his mother said, her grief worn down by the retelling and by time. "It was as if he had his own self-constructed ostomy. He was so traumatized by the first ostomy, he was afraid that he would go back into the hospital and end up with another one. He couldn't deal with that. I think he wanted to force them to do the transplant. There was no way he was going to listen to me or anybody else. The fistula hemorrhaged, and he was bleeding externally."

The night before Gideon was scheduled to fly to a Los Angeles medical center to be evaluated for an intestinal transplant, he bled to death, alone in his apartment. He was 26.

"I remember reading an article when Gideon was a teenager written by a man who mentioned that his wife had died of Crohn's disease," said Linda. "I remember at that time that I said to my therapist, 'I didn't know people died of Crohn's,' and it terrified me. I never asked the doctor about it. My approach was: What can he do so he can get better and go into remission?"

Focusing on mortality rates doesn't help patients to live their lives with IBD from a stance of perseverance and optimism. The statistics are meaningless. The reality is that most people with IBD live a normal lifetime, despite surgeries, medications, and all. But if the example of someone who died because he didn't seek care fast enough is sufficiently chilling, it may motivate patients to take their symptoms seriously and attend to their illness as if their life depended on it.

CHAPTER THIRTEEN
IBD Camps Change Lives

When you think about a camp that caters to children with IBD, it's easy to imagine a sad refuge for sickly individuals who stagger from one discussion group to another and whose identity centers around their Crohn's disease or ulcerative colitis. Kathy said her son had wondered, "'Why would I want to sit around and talk about my disease with other sick kids?'"

Nothing could be further from the reality. Camps designed for kids with IBD are like any other camp, except that they provide a different kind of experience, an experience of being fully known. "You don't have to explain," Isabelle said. "People get it."

The young people I interviewed who attended such camps came back with glowing reviews. They'd made life-long friends, as one does in any sleep-away camp, but with a twist. These friends understood what each other had been through and they didn't have to hide their condition. None of them had to justify why they took a fistful of pills several times a day.

Two camp systems in North America have been created to provide children and adolescents with a setting that is at once relaxed and active, and where campers do not need to explain their IBD symptoms or treatment. They are Camp Oasis in the United States, run by the CCFA, and the Crohn's and Colitis Youth Camp in Canada, run by Crohn's and Colitis Canada. The counselors have IBD and the counselor-to-camper ratio is 1:6. The social workers and psychologists on staff either have IBD themselves or they have extensive experience in working with kids with IBD.

Sarah, who began going to Camp Oasis at age 13, two years after she was diagnosed with Crohn's disease, found that "being surrounded by people who understood made it easier to feel open about it. I used to be really shy. I've been there seven summers. It's given me a lot of really good friends. It was really cool. At every meal, every table has a huge bin of each kid's medicine. There are four seats reserved for boxes of medications. Then we'd have a competition [about who can swallow the most pills at once]. I can swallow eight pills at one time," she said proudly, and then she turned serious. "I don't have the most severe case. There would be kids who'd have feeding tubes at night and talk about staying in the hospital. It made you realize that if the people around you can be so strong, you should be able to do it."

Other than the dispensing of medications, you wouldn't know this was a camp for kids with Crohn's disease and ulcerative colitis. When I visited a Camp Oasis in upstate New York, kids were busy with activities typical at any camp: drawing, painting, music, drama, dance, soccer, tennis, baseball, scavenger hunts, orienteering, map making, compass usage, hiking, exploring science in nature, swimming and a ropes course. A 50-minute rest period during the day gives campers the chance to talk with a gastroenterologist and ask questions that they may have not been able to ask while in their own doctor's office.

When Clinton was sick with Crohn's disease at a Canadian children's hospital, nurses encouraged him to go to the Crohn's and Colitis Youth Camp in Alberta. Clinton refused. "Clinton at first just wanted to go back to school to be a normal kid," said his mother, Wendy. "The disease had taken him over for so long, he wanted to be around his friends, do what teenagers do and have a good time. I tried to convince him to go. About ten days before camp, he suddenly said, 'I'm going to go.' He later said he cried when he went and he cried when he had to leave. It was a really positive experience for him." Clinton said that camp "really helped me come to terms with my ostomy and helped me meet other people."

Colin started at Camp Oasis in Michigan, not as a camper but as a counselor. "It's just an amazing experience, he said. "They run into all these kids their own age they can talk to and later 'friend' on Facebook. Some of the counselors got together with the older campers, who are 15 and 16, and invited them to ask us questions, like what's it like to go to college with the disease," Colin continued. "What's it like being an adult with the disease? We tell them that you can go to college and be fine. Or you can be out of college in the working world and be fine. No matter how bad it seems in high school, it gets better."

Kevin, who was diagnosed with Crohn's disease at age 9, said he liked being in a place "where people your own age know exactly what you're talking about. I had never told people about my Crohn's, because I didn't want them to have sympathy for me. I didn't want them to think I needed special treatment. But at camp, you can tell them anything, because they wouldn't look at you any differently than if you didn't have the disease. My friends at camp are down-to-earth people. We're all there to have a good time and there's no drama because we don't worry or let things bother us."

An obstacle to deciding whether to go to an IBD camp is the perception that your disease isn't so bad and that the camp is really for people who have a serious case. You may reason that your condition is so mild you don't belong there.

When Kathleen went to Camp Oasis, she was convinced she didn't have Crohn's at all anymore, until her mother explained that she was in remission. "I was really skeptical at first," Kathleen said. "I couldn't see how it could be fun at all. But I agreed and went. It was amazing just to see how many other kids there were just like me. It gave me perspective to help other kids who were on steroids and all puffed up or had surgeries. It was eye opening for me. It's for any kids with Crohn's and colitis. There was a real range of kids there."

Jesse first went to Camp Oasis at age 9, a month after he had undergone a total colectomy for runaway ulcerative colitis and started wearing an ostomy bag. "Normally I would not have let him go," said his mother, Amy. "I was kind of a basket case, and my husband was also kind of freaked out, and his response was to give Jesse whatever he wanted. When Jesse said he wanted to go to camp, I had no fight in me. He'll probably be going until he's a counselor."

Jonathan also decided to go to Camp Oasis at age 9, first as a camper, and he returned every year until he was 19, when he was a counselor. "It was awesome," he said. "All my friends with Crohn's disease are from that place. Camp showed me that you can just joke about it. The kids were relaxed. Their attitude was, we're going to live with it. The friends I made there, I still talk with to this day, because every kid has at least one thing in common. We all have Crohn's or colitis. Even if we may not like the same things, we all have something we can talk about, but the best part of going there was that nobody talked about it. We all knew why we were there; we all knew why we got in. There was no reason to bring it up. That put people closer together."

Nicole, who went at age 13, also enjoyed the fact that "it was a regular sleep-away camp: You woke up at 7, went to breakfast, went to the canteen where you'd sing, went back to the bunk, did some activities, had lunch, more zip-lining, crafts, cooking, pool, tubing in the lake, jet ski, activities, a scavenger hunt or a dance. No programming around the disease. You'd make great friendships with other people like you."

Campers with Crohn's disease call each other "Crohnies" (there doesn't seem to be a nickname for ulcerative colitis) and then there is everybody else — that is, people who do not have IBD. Camp provides an opportunity to feel on top. "When we talk about everyone else," Nicole said, "we roll our eyes, because a lot of people don't understand that just because it's a gross disease, we're still normal people functioning very well in society. I went into it a little skeptical and I couldn't be happier.

"I remember one summer," she said, "there was also a karate camp at our host camp and someone told them we were a disease camp. They all panicked and thought we were contagious. So, we tortured them. We'd be in the pool and they didn't want to come in. If I'd been at home, I would have been mortified, but because we were an army, it was the funniest thing in the world."

Kids Who Say No to Camp

Despite the accolades from campers and parents, a number of young people reported that they had decided against attending an IBD camp, not wanting to define themselves by their disease.

Scott, whose Crohn's disease was so serious that he had taken Prednisone for a decade, "didn't want to affiliate or recognize himself as having that illness," his mother said. Scott told me, "I was not going to go to camp. I didn't want to talk about it. I didn't want to deal with it. By college, I didn't have anybody I could turn to, to talk about the issue."

Phil, who had two abscesses, a fistula, and a bowel resection after being diagnosed with Crohn's at 16, said he "thought it was silly to define myself so essentially in that way. I saw no reason to kind of amplify the role it played in my life. Everybody's got their thing. I viewed having Crohn's like having asthma or being lactose intolerant. It's an ailment people have to live with." Phil, who is Jewish, added, "You go to Jewish camp. You don't go to Crohn's and colitis camp."

Those who have attended disagree. "It's a shame that someone would turn down an opportunity to go there," said Colin. "If someone has a child with the disease, I'd find a way to enroll them in the camp. It's a week for the kids just to water ski, climb rock walls, canoe, and escape from their lives."

Ostomy Camp

Although some kids at Camp Oasis wear ostomy bags, there are two specialized camps for kids with ostomies — Youth Rally in Colorado and the Ostomy Canada Youth Camp near Calgary, Canada.

Krystal, who is Canadian, first went to the youth camp when she was 9. "I didn't even know how to change my bag on my own yet," she said. "It was a really great experience. I remember feeling sorry for myself and having a lot of 'Why me?' days before going to camp. I still have them, but at camp it was the first time ever meeting someone who had Crohn's and an ostomy. I had gone to an ostomy [support group] meeting where I live, but it was all elderly people. There were no kids, and I didn't think there was anybody else my age who had an ostomy. At this camp, there are all these other kids having fun."

Krystal returned every year as a camper, and when I talked to her, she was working there as a counselor. "I'd be a completely different person if I didn't go to camp," Krystal told me. "I have a whole camp family — a camp mom and camp friends I talk to as often as I can. It's such a great support system. Everyone has a different story of telling friends on the outside and coming to the point of acceptance. I came back a completely different kid."

Conclusion

This book has been deliberately non-prescriptive. Its purpose is to lay out the ways people with IBD function in their daily lives and how they navigate their way through obstacles. However, observing life at IBD camps and listening to people talk about them tempts me to offer one piece of advice: Go. Sign up. Try it. It's only one week at the end of summer. You'll love it.

CHAPTER FOURTEEN
Dating, Intimacy, and Marriage

> I really don't think I'm ready to date yet! As you might imagine, I'm a little self-conscious about my leaky anus to try and fumble with getting a woman's bra off. I just can't do it, can't do it, can't get involved with a woman intimately. Really, it's just too much work, too much hassle, too much anxiety.
>
> — *A Recluse's Guide*
> **by Ben Brandfon (unpublished novel)**

The Joke

I told a joke to everyone of dating age I interviewed to ease the transition into talking about the intimate and very personal area of dating and sex. I offer it here because I think it's funny and because sometimes IBD can be so sad that laughing is a healthy outlet. I have a strong hunch that the author of this joke either had IBD or was in relationship with someone who did:

Three engineers were discussing the nature of God. The first said, "When you consider the complex structure of the skeleton and the muscles, it's obvious that God must be a mechanical engineer." Said the second: "No. The thing that makes a human being human is the brain and nervous system. When you consider all the electrical signals that must be transmitted and processed, it's clear that God is an electrical engineer" Third guy: "You're both wrong. Only a civil engineer would put a waste disposal pipeline right through a recreational area."

Who thinks about the proximity of the anus to the sexual organs? Only people who experience pain and cramping, leaking during sex, loud noises in the bathroom, and smelly smells. That is, people with IBD. For them, navigating the world of dating and intimacy can feel like running through a minefield.

Finding Someone to Trust

To find a compatible partner is challenging under the best of circumstances, and it often entails serendipity. What further complicates dating and intimacy is the quest to find someone whom you trust to tell about your IBD, someone who will tolerate not only the gas and smells, but also the frequent and interminable trips to the bathroom, the fatigue, the need to leave parties early, the constraints on drinking and eating, and the fact that all these realities will ebb and flow throughout your lifetime.

If you do encounter a romantic partner you trust enough to love you through seemingly shameful and vulnerable moments, the relationship can feel like a sanctuary and a refuge. Although IBD can delay dating and intimacy when patients are in the grip of humiliation and embarrassment, most of the people I interviewed found that once they overcame their reluctance to open up about their condition and treat their bodily functions as part of the human experience, the right partner offered acceptance and almost endless patience.

First, though, people with IBD have to overcome being emotionally immobilized in order to thrust themselves into the dating world.

Inhibitions

Monica's romantic life has long been paralyzed by her fears about what a man would say about the smells and noises she makes when she is in the bathroom. Diagnosed with ulcerative colitis at age 15, she had J-pouch surgery at 22 and she has spent the years since alone. "I'm not married. I've had very few intimate relationships because I don't want to have to share that part with somebody," she said. "It's embarrassing. What if I have a leakage at night, which as I get older becomes every once in a while? What if I fart at night? When I'm sleeping, I don't have control. When I go to the bathroom, I have a lot of gas. You can hear it. If I were not so self-conscious, maybe I wouldn't feel that way."

Although Monica feels more inhibited than most, she is not alone. Kevin, who was diagnosed at 15, also had a rocky time with relationships. The girlfriend he dated for five years in high school and college "couldn't take me having Crohn's, with the frequent bathroom visits. It was hard to be intimate with her, because I had an ostomy. She just left. After that, there's always a big fear that the next person will get tired and not want to deal with it."

Kevin is honest about his fear of rejection. "It's hard to find somebody to feel comfortable with, so that even if an accident happens, you know they're not going to treat you any different." After a failed marriage, he has a steady girlfriend, and now, Crohn's is openly a part of who he is.

It is striking that both Monica and Kevin were diagnosed at 15, when romantic feelings begin to bloom in earnest. Their self-confidence and their sense of a normal self seem to have been suspended in a time of uncertainty and emotional disturbance, a time from which they have recovered slowly or not at all.

Coming Right Out with It

Some people with IBD have no misgivings about speaking frankly about their illness. Stephanie, 28, who was diagnosed at age 10, never flinched about telling her date right from the outset that she has serious ulcerative colitis. Divorced and taking care of a small child, she had no room for someone who wouldn't accept her disease. "Before I even started dating someone, I made sure he knew," she said. Her mother asked why she was so quick to be open. Stephanie reasoned that if she had a flare-up and her boyfriend didn't know how to take care of her, the relationship wouldn't work. If he didn't *want* to take care of her, she said, "He's not the right person for me." Stephanie acknowledges her colitis as a major part of her life and believes that it must be accepted by anyone she's with.

Some young people with IBD achieve a comfort level with fairly new romantic partners, acting as if they were long married. Tatiana, 19, whose Crohn's was caught early and was under reasonable control, said that if she has to make a lengthy visit to the bathroom, "I'll tell him I'm going to go poop. Later, he'll ask me, 'Is it a crummy poop?' If it is, he'll say, 'Okay, I'll stay away from the bathroom for a while.'"

Most of the time, communication between Tatiana and her boyfriend was good. One time, however, tension arose over just how urgently she needed a bathroom. They were driving 45 minutes from her home, and Tatiana was ready to knock on any door and plead to use the bathroom. Her boyfriend said she could hold it. She begged him to pull over, but when he refused, she forced herself to hold it until she got home. He turned out to be right, but she said, "It was the worse day I've had."

Nicole, 18, who was diagnosed with ulcerative colitis at age 9, has dated boys who have IBD and boys who have never heard of it. She met her first boyfriend at Camp Oasis, the one-week summer camp for young people with IBD. "We've all been really close over the years," she said of her fellow campers. "Everyone's kind of inter-dated, because there's a sense of understanding when you don't have to explain to someone you're dating that you get stomach aches and have to go to the bathroom. It saves so much time and hassle."

Since then, Nicole has dated people who don't know about the disease and, she said, "It was weird. It was hard to explain it to them," although, she conceded, as she's gotten a little older, most young men she meets have been understanding when she tells them about her ulcerative colitis. "The general consensus is that everyone has something," she said. "Nobody's perfect. I'm sure the person I'm dating has some issue they do or don't want to talk about. I usually take their reaction to me with a grain of salt. There have been times when they've been skeptical, but no one's ever told me, 'I don't want to date you anymore because you have this disease.'"

Ostomies and Romance

Rachel, 25, who was diagnosed at age 13, was similarly frank with her boyfriend, whom she'd met on the Internet just before she had a serious Crohn's flare. She made a deliberate decision to change the way she had behaved with earlier boyfriends. "In the past, I've broken up with people rather than tell them what was wrong with me," she said. "I've pushed people away instead of letting them get close to me."

This time, she acted differently. "He didn't understand what I was going through until recently, when I decided to start talking with him about it, even the most embarrassing moments," she said. "Now he really understands what I go through on a day-to-day basis."

After the frank conversation, Rachel's boyfriend consulted the Internet about Crohn's disease. "It was a big mistake," she said drily. "He came across horror stories. I had to sit him down and say, 'No, no, that's not going to happen.' Then he was finding miracle cures online. He'd say, 'Why don't you try this?' I'd tell him, 'No. That won't work.'"

Rachel found that no matter how sick she became, "I couldn't get rid of him." This is not to say he wasn't distressed. "He's not used to illness," she said. "He's never had anything wrong with him, never spent any time in a hospital. So, since he's been with me, I think he's seen more illness, pain, and suffering than he can cope with. He found it very hard, indeed, because I had a lot of complications."

Since her ostomy surgery nine months earlier, Rachel hadn't been sexually intimate with her boyfriend. "Everything hurts, and the last thing you want to do is to make the pain worse," she said. "I'm amazed he stuck with me. He says he'll be patient until I'm ready to be intimate again. I really don't know when I'll be ready. I'm avoiding sex as much as possible. I'm not at my most attractive. I think that's the most difficult thing as a woman with Crohn's. Even if you look okay, you feel disgusting."

Parents' Fears and Hopes

Behind the scenes, most parents of a young person who falls in love with someone with IBD stand back and worry as the relationship flowers. Will their child's ill partner fully function as a spouse and parent or will he or she be dependent throughout the marriage?

Bob, who was diagnosed at age 11, is now married with two children. He is a vice-president of a major financial firm. He said that when he met the woman he would later marry, "I was 29 and, for two thirds of that time, I was in and out of the hospital. I think she had reservations, like anybody would. She overcame them." Her parents were not so sure. "They wanted to make sure she was taken care of. They had a fear she would marry someone who might not be able to provide for her." Bob understands his in-laws' concerns. "They're wonderful people. It's their daughter. I'd have concerns for my children if they fell in love with somebody with Crohn's."

The parents of the young person with IBD also have fears and hopes for their child's relationship. They hope the person whom their child marries will have the fortitude and desire to care for the sick partner during down times. Laura, for example, crossed her fingers when her son, Thomas, who wears an ostomy bag and has serious Crohn's disease, began a relationship with a young woman Laura liked very much. "This girl is phenomenal," she said, explaining that the young woman has a nursing degree and is able to take care of Thomas' medical needs. "I pray every day it isn't going to freak her out, that she isn't going to look at his bag and say, 'Oh, I see you had asparagus last night.' She hasn't been grossed out by it. So far, he has maintained that relationship. He's terrified that if they ever do break up — how he will tell the next girl about his Crohn's? I say, 'Let's cross that bridge if we come to it.' This girl suffered through not going to the college parties everyone was going to. He's been very blessed."

Feeling Sexual

Betsy, 24, who was diagnosed with Crohn's disease at age 11, didn't date much in college. "I was a major prude," she said. "I was embarrassed and didn't want to get into that situation with someone I didn't know very well." A few months before our interview, Betsy began to date Andrew, whom she trusted enough to tell about her Crohn's almost at the outset. "I just felt really close to him. It's a big part of me, and he needed to know." It turned out that Andrew's best friend's girlfriend also has Crohn's, and he knew all about it. Despite his positive response, Betsy still is self-conscious about the smells and noise she makes in the bathroom and she takes steps to avoid exposing him to them.

"Feeling sexual can be tricky," she said. "I can tell him if I'm not feeling well, but I don't go in his toilet at all. I go upstairs if we're downstairs and downstairs if we're upstairs. Maybe he knows it, but we haven't talked about it. If we're out, I'll go before we go home, or after him before we go to bed. I'll have gas when we go to bed, and so we sleep with the fan on. It creates white noise, and keeps the air moving."

At one point, Betsy added, Andrew "ran the idea of anal sex by me. I told him, 'No way. I have inflammatory bowel disease.' He realized it was a mistake and said, 'Never mind, never mind. It was dumb.'" Andrew recognizes that when Betsy isn't feeling well, she gets into a darker mood. "I'm her partner. I want to lighten her load," he said. "When she's feeling like that, I do some of the chores to ease her burden, so she can lie down and feel comfortable. That's my biggest role, to make her as comfortable as she can be when she's feeling bad. Nobody wants to feel like that, but it's okay that she feels bad. It sucks, but if she knows that I'm okay with it, then she doesn't feel like she needs to be 'on' all the time."

Dating and Committed

I had been dating Jake for four years when I got the news that I would need a total colectomy. Before that, I was in remission, so my ulcerative colitis didn't interfere with our relationship, except that I needed to swallow a tall glass of gelatinous psyllium seed at bedtime and take medication three times a day ~ not very sexy.

But Jake said he fell in love with me even more deeply as he watched me take responsibility for the decision to undergo the surgery and then handle the surgery itself. He asked me if I wanted to get a second opinion and I reacted almost fiercely. It was my body, I told him, and it was my decision to do what I needed to do. He fed me ice chips after surgery. He emailed my friends and acquaintances about my condition. I, in turn, told him which street was safer to walk on late at night from the hospital, garbling my words while still under the effects of lingering anesthesia. He thought that was amazing. Less than two years later, we married.

The pressures created by IBD can make or break a relationship. There are many elements that have nothing to do with IBD that can affect two people as they decide whether to commit to each other, but IBD presents special challenges, given that they are life long.

Alan, who graduated from the University of Colorado in Boulder, was diagnosed with Crohn's disease during his senior year of college, after years of being misdiagnosed and suffering with symptoms. He told his girlfriend, Ellie, about the diagnosis on the phone. "It was really hard for me to tell her, because I was feeling bad that she had to put up with it. She said it didn't matter. She just wanted to help me to get through it. She was always there when I was sick. It is the only thing anyone can do — be there. It really helps."

David, who was diagnosed at age 11, works for a consulting firm in New York, and at 25, he has long hid the pain and discomfort of his Crohn's disease. He drinks alcohol socially, which many people with Crohn's avoid, and as a consequence, he will occasionally leave a party early, go home, and crawl into bed in a fetal position until the pain subsides. He would rather feel the pain than stand out.

David has dated Kathy for four years, after being good friends for four years, giving the relationship a solid foundation. Kathy learned about his Crohn's early in their friendship. However, she said, "It wasn't a big reveal. It was casually mentioned. He said, 'Hey, I can't eat this carrot.' I asked him why not. 'I have Crohn's.' I said, 'What's that?' I didn't become aware that it was something he had to think about on a regular basis until we were dating."

David was concerned that if he talked openly about his Crohn's, people would treat him differently. He had become adept at acting normal. "He doesn't want to be perceived as weak, even though he wouldn't be," Kathy said. "He would leave a party if he were feeling symptoms, rather than sit down and say, 'Hold on a minute,' and deal with people asking questions.

"Once we started dating, maybe he thought he could open up more," she said. "Or maybe I forced him to open up, because I was around all the time, but he said I was the first person outside his family he'd allow to see him in pain. That was when I realized this is kind of serious." That was six months into their dating life, four-and-a-half years after they'd met.

Kathy now takes her cues from David. He doesn't have severe episodes often, and when he does, she knows not to fuss over him. She said that Crohn's has affected their life together minimally or not at all, but as she continued to talk, she recounted a handful of times when they went home early from a bar or a party because David wasn't feeling well. "I have seen him doubled over," she said. "He tends to lie down and curl up. He does a lot of abdominal massage for himself. It cuts short our social time or maybe we won't go to some event we had planned on going to."

Having sex in a way that doesn't hurt the person with IBD is especially relevant to gay men. I spoke with only two gay men with Crohn's disease, although I tried to find others without success. Both men said that they avoid anal intercourse and find other ways to have intimate relations. Morty, Jerry's partner for 10 years, was 21 when they met and he didn't know about Jerry's Crohn's for almost a year. He is voluble about how much he wants to be involved and caring during the ups and downs of Jerry's disease, and he complains that Jerry sometimes feels intruded upon.

The irony is that Morty, the healthy one, has considerable shame about the smells he makes. "Before we met, I had never actually passed gas in front of someone," Morty said. "I was freaked out that someone might know I had this toxic stuff inside me. With Jerry, I'd never smelled something so strong. I thought it was strange that he was so okay with it and didn't seem to feel the shame I felt. I remember allowing myself to pass gas in our bed and thinking something huge had shifted for me. I felt such acceptance. I felt like I could be with someone who wouldn't sweat the small things because of all of his history. I know now that Jerry had had a lot of shame about Crohn's and his body. But it took several years before I could see any of that."

Marriage

The complexity that exists in every couple's relationship is certainly intensified by the nuances of IBD and intimacy, as exemplified by the experience of Susan and Charles. They met during her freshman year of college, two years before she was diagnosed with ulcerative colitis. In college, they had an active sex life, even after her diagnosis.

After she graduated, they married, and their sex life went south when her ulcerative colitis intensified. "When I'm having a stomach ache at night or if I'm not feeling good mentally or I don't feel sexy or I'm bloated, it's really hard for me to have sexual intercourse," she said. "Obviously, that poses a problem, especially because we were having sex every day in college. I've worked on this a lot in therapy and have figured out a way to please my husband and have sexual relations without having intercourse and not feeling guilty."

Susan understands that her reluctance has put a strain on their relationship. "I don't want our relationship to go to s—-," she said. "We do have sex, but it's not all the time. How can I have sex? It hurts. It's not a good thing. I'm 27 and the terms have changed."

Charles thinks that Susan doesn't have as strong a sex drive as he does, and that she uses her disease to avoid being intimate. He acknowledges that there are times when she does feel ill. However, he contends that she doesn't communicate well, so he feels rejected. "It's definitely an adjustment," he said. "She wants to be Debbie Downer and say, 'I'm not feeling good.' The only issue for me is when she doesn't communicate. She'll reject me and won't state why.

"She doesn't want to say, 'I've got stomach issues.' She felt she was being repetitive and didn't want me to see that her colitis had such a bad effect on our sexual life," Charles continued. "She wasn't really rejecting me. A lot of times, emotional issues cause a flare-up. Even if she eats something that doesn't sit well with her, it can affect our whole evening together. It's partially food, partially emotional, partially her ulcerative colitis, which is not nearly as bad as it once was."

Gillian and her husband, Hugo, had an impasse over her temporary ostomy. "My husband couldn't look at it. It bothered him," she said. "It makes funny noises, which is funny when you're trying to be romantic," she said. "It can gurgle and start puffing up if I had gassy foods. My biggest problem with it was seeing the bag when we were trying to do anything. That was a mood killer, so I'd get those skimpy tank tops that are very stretchy. I'd wear those and they would hold everything in and support my stomach a little, too. That made it a little easier."

Hugo decided to see a counselor for couple's therapy, "because you end up having fights," he said. He said he is grateful to the CCFA after attending a group session and listening to other people talk about their struggles. He advised: "Don't be afraid to ask for professional advice about relationship issues. You need somebody else to tell you what you already know or help you through it."

Wish List

The decision about whom to marry is probably the most important decision in life, more important than what college or graduate school you will attend or what career you will undertake. Choosing a partner will determine the course of your life. Whether you are the partner with IBD or the partner who will care for someone with IBD, there are certain qualities that are necessary to make a good match that will last.

Rose summed up what many of the people with IBD whom I interviewed said they wanted from a mate. Acknowledging that her ulcerative colitis has interfered with her sexual desire, she said her condition has made her seek out certain people and judge them by whether they can handle her illness.

"I'm looking for someone who's compassionate and understanding, who shows me they're attracted to me no matter what," she said. "My last boyfriend was really open about it and made me feel I was definitely desired. Even when we weren't able to have sex, it was still okay. I want someone who's not going to baby me and worry constantly and someone who will learn about my disease, so I'm not constantly isolated with it. I'd like someone to make it lighter when it's happening. When I'm feeling serious, I'd like someone to make the situation less heavy."

When you are married, you hope that the vow "for better or for worse" will kick in. The commitment to work out whatever comes along creates a feeling of stability. However, when IBD gets worse after your marriage, the issues that arise are difficult to grapple with, especially when it comes to sexual intimacy. When partners come to an impasse, seeking help from a counselor is a healthy way to break through.

Among those interviewed, spouses' reactions ranged from being understanding and endlessly patient to being repulsed and squeamish. IBD patients sometimes felt bad that when they fell ill, they could not be attuned to their healthy partner's needs. Partners with IBD also don't want to sound like a broken record every time they turn their partner down. Healthy partners want to know that they aren't being rejected — rather, that the illness is keeping intimacy at bay. Enduring love may be tested by the strictures imposed by IBD, but, all other things being equal, love need not break down under the pressures of IBD.

Below you will find resources for information and advice to help you through the challenges of a close, intimate relationship.

- The United Ostomy Associations of America (UOA) has published excellent brochures about sexuality and sexual function. For example: "Sex, Courtship and the Single Ostomate," "Sex and the Female Ostomate," "Sex and the Male Ostomate," and "Gay and Lesbian Ostomates and their Caregivers." Although written for people with ostomies, the information on sexual function, relationships, and body image will serve anyone with IBD very well. You can find these brochures on the Web by title or at www.uoa.org.
- The CCFA offers information about sex and IBD at www.ccfa.org/resources/sex-and-ibd.html
- You can contact the American Association of Sexuality Educators, Counselors and Therapists at P.O. Box 238, Mount Vernon, Iowa 52314 or by email, at AASECT@worldnet.att.net.

CHAPTER FIFTEEN
Siblings

How is the healthy sibling of someone with IBD affected by the illness? What is the emotional legacy when parents are focused on getting IBD under control and the healthy sibling feels left out? How much information is it advisable to give to a sibling about a brother or sister's health status? How do parents deal with the dynamics between their healthy and sick children?

I asked these questions out of ignorance. I have no siblings. I have never felt jealousy, love, concern, or competitiveness from a contemporary in my family, nor had those feelings intensify when I was sick. However, what I have heard from mental health professionals and from siblings of people with IBD has helped me to understand the complexities of the issues families face and, particularly, the bind healthy siblings find themselves in.

Importance of Sibling Relationships

Let's first establish the strong influence of sibling relationships on all areas of life. Whether one is in sickness or in health, the primacy of one's sibling relationships throughout life is too often overlooked. More than 82 percent of people under 18 in the United States live with at least one sibling. (McHale, 2012) That's more than the number of children who live with a father in the home. "The relationship between siblings lasts longer than with parents," pointed out Dr. Debra Lobato, director of child psychology at Rhode Island Hospital and Hasbro Children's Hospital in Providence, R.I. and a professor at the Warren Alpert Medical School of Brown University. "For siblings not to be acknowledged as important is to ignore a really major part of life."

When a sibling is ill with IBD, the connection with healthy siblings can be filled with ambivalence and complexity. "Conflicted, guilty, resentful," are some of the emotions that healthy siblings may feel toward their sick sibling, according to Dr. Karen Gail Lewis, a psychologist in the Cincinnati and Washington, D.C. areas who has worked with siblings for more than 40 years.

"They feel ambivalence," she said of the healthy siblings' attitude toward their sick brother or sister. "I love my sibling. I hate my sibling. I love my parents. I hate them." These feelings may at first seem like garden-variety emotional swings found in every household, but when a sibling is sick with IBD and parents are distracted and pulled toward the sick sibling, the healthy ones may feel that they don't have the right to express negative emotions, Dr. Lewis said. They often repress emotions that even they can't identify. In addition, problems arise when the healthy sibling gets the subtle message that "nothing that I need will be as important as what my sick sibling needs," she said. Dr. Lobato said of the healthy sibling, "I see as much resentment of the parents as of the sick kid. Who's their champion?"

If healthy siblings feel neglected, they may seem oblivious to their sibling's illness or they may act in more overtly negative ways. For their part, sick siblings often notice the inattention and remember it years later, just as they remember healthy siblings who were kind and loving. Sometimes, the edges between the healthy siblings' two responses to the illness may blur.

"I know my sister was worried, and she didn't know how to deal with the situation," said Alyssa, 24, of her older, healthy sister, Erica. "She spent a lot of time with her friends and buried herself in her schoolwork because of it."

Erica didn't see it that way. Her mother, she said, "needed to focus on Alyssa. I didn't feel neglected. I was working, doing all my activities, going to school. Alyssa needed her more. If I needed my mom at that time, she would have been there for me. I wasn't sick."

According to the scenario that Dr. Lewis describes, Erica may, indeed, have loved Alyssa and not wanted to call attention away from her. A healthy sibling like this becomes "a hidden kid who doesn't speak up for her needs." As adults, such siblings may become people pleasers and caretakers, according to Dr. Lewis. While they're being good and understanding and feeling worried about their siblings and parents, they also worry about being regarded as selfish. They may think, "'If I want to go shopping with Mom and now she can't go because my sister is sick, I shouldn't be so selfish that I feel bad or even resentful,'" the psychologist said. "There's no one telling the healthy sibling that it's okay to have those feelings."

Dr. Lobato observed that there are problems even when parents spend time with the healthy sibling. "If they answer complaints with, 'What if you had to have needles like your brother?' or, 'Think of all the medical procedures you don't have to go through because you're not sick,' the message is that the healthy sibling's feelings are not valid," she said. "If the parent defends the greater attention they give to the child with the illness and try to use logic with the healthy siblings and tell them all the reasons they should not feel badly, that further alienates the siblings from each other."

Dr. Lobato suggested a better approach: "Instead, parents can acknowledge the healthy siblings' feelings in the moment without judging them and then communicate that they understand that it's sometimes hard for siblings, too — that IBD affects not just the kid who has it, but everyone in the family. Then resentment will diminish. If the parent says to the sibling, 'Maybe sometimes you feel a little bit jealous,' all the wind comes out of the resentment. The child knows the parent understands and can move on." She also suggested that in families where the healthy siblings take on extra chores and tasks, their effort should be verbally acknowledged and appreciated.

Dr. Lobato's study found a continuum of behaviors on the part of healthy siblings that ranged from support of their sick brother or sister all the way to sabotage. Helpful siblings call their sick sibling in the hospital and "maintain some contact with [the sick sibling] to keep their spirits up," she said. "They will show discretion. They do not talk about bathroom problems with peers and they maintain privacy. If the sick child doesn't want their IBD to be talked about, the siblings adhere to that. They take on more chores. They step up and do some of the brother or sister's work. And they give them extra time in the bathroom."

Healthy siblings who sabotage their relationship with the sick sibling "complain about the condition of the bathroom and that they had to pick up the brother or sister's homework from school," Dr. Lobato said. "My belief is the relationship was poor to begin with and the IBD gives them something they can complain about. If you have a bad relationship, there will be more sabotage, but if you have a good relationship, it's very helpful" to the sibling with IBD.

Joseph and his stepbrother embodied a broken relationship. During Joseph's freshman year of high school, his stepbrother spread a story around school that Joseph had undergone a colonoscopy and had a scope up his butt. "Everybody began making fun of me," Joseph said. This "gotcha" created a short-lived social victory for Joseph's brother at the expense of Joseph's self-confidence.

Parents' and Siblings' Distress

"My parents made rules that they said were immoveable, but they changed them for David," said Sheila, more than a decade after her 11-year-old brother was diagnosed with Crohn's disease when she was 15. "I felt resentment. My parents refused to let us have video games, but for David they offered, 'We'll get you this game, we'll get you that game.' That was one incident that led to a big blowup. Then David got hamsters and other things I couldn't have."

The stress on parents when a healthy sibling is at war with the sick one cannot be underestimated. David and Sheila's mother, Cathy, still has a painful memory of her healthy adolescent daughter showering antagonism onto her sick brother and onto her and her husband.

"Sheila was the star in our family, the first born, and David was born four years later," Cathy said. "Then, all of a sudden, David got sick. Suddenly, the attention shifted to David, and Sheila was jealous. She threw a tantrum, saying David was faking it and it wasn't real. It was hard, really hard. I remember being angry with her — not a very proud moment on my part — but it was such a scary time. Here was my daughter being a kid about it, being a pain in the ass, being jealous and angry and provocative."

Sheila and David, now both in their 20s, live in different cities and don't see each other much, but they get along. Sheila feels that her complaints and tantrums were aimed more at her parents than at her brother. "I don't think I resented him," she said. "I was scared because my brother was sick, but my parents bending the rules for him — that bothered me."

Dr. Kodman-Jones, a psychologist who has long experience working with families of IBD children, said that healthy siblings "feel kind of invisible. Parents give the sick kid the extra-special things, like a computer, and the other sibling is, like, 'Wait a minute. I'm a senior. He's just a sophomore.' They're sensitive to the way parental decisions are made."

Long-lasting Resentment

Sometimes, jealousy that begins over the attention given to a sick sibling doesn't heal even when the siblings get older. Krystal, 18, believes that her 16-year-old sister "felt left out a lot" when they were younger. Their mother frequently stayed with her in the hospital when she was terribly sick, Krystal said, adding, "My sister wouldn't see my mom at all. She'd stay at my grandparents' house if my dad came to the hospital. And I'd get all kinds of presents every time I went into the hospital. At family functions, I'd be the one who was asked how I was. She probably felt as if she were in the background of a lot of things.

"We used to fight about it a lot," Krystal continued. "She'd get jealous because I'd have all these new toys. I didn't want any of those toys and didn't want to be in this position for all these presents. We fought over attention, regular sister things. We aren't close today."

Few Studies on Sibling relationships

Given the complexity of the relationship between healthy siblings and young people with IBD, it's surprising how few studies have examined these issues. Although Western medicine has become more sophisticated about the connection between mental health and medical illness, major funding institutions are still reluctant to apply their limited dollars to exploring the issues faced by healthy siblings.

Indeed, the numbers of siblings interviewed for the few studies that have been done is almost absurdly small. Only three studies, examining 20 siblings or fewer, have been published, and two of them date back to the 1990s. The studies were nonetheless informative.

In one of the studies, Swedish researcher Ingemar Engstrom studied 20 healthy siblings of patients with IBD between the ages of 7 and 18. He found that their self-esteem was lower, and their levels of anxiety and depression were higher than were those of healthy siblings of patients with any other chronic illness. (Engstrom, 1992)

The reasons for this were explained by a group of English researchers led by Dr. Anthony K. Akobeng, a pediatric gastroenterologist. Although the researchers interviewed only seven siblings, they came up with a wide range of concerns. The siblings "worry about the sick child's having to go into the hospital and about the long-term effects of the disease and its treatment on their brother or sister," the researchers reported. "Some siblings resent that they are made to do many more household chores than their ill sibling. They are jealous because of the special treatment and constant attention that the ill child receives from the parents. There may be times when they feel neglected by the parents." (Akobeng, 1999)

Some siblings were worried about their ill brother or sister being bullied at school because of their appearance (weight gain from steroids or weight loss from their disease). And, significantly, healthy siblings felt that their parents were secretive about their brother or sister's illness and tried to keep them in the dark.

Carly's brother was such a sibling. He was 6 when Carly went into the hospital, and "he felt I got all the attention," she said. Her parents would "send him to my aunts and grandparents for sleepovers. My parents thought he was having fun, but he felt left out because he didn't know what was going on. He was staying at other people's houses when he wanted to be with our family. And when he saw me again, I looked sicker than before, and he didn't understand why. I think he knew some of it, but he didn't feel he knew enough."

Washington-area psychologist Dr. Karen Lewis thinks that parents should give younger, healthy children as much information as they think the child can handle. In fact, she added, "The kid may be able to handle a lot more than the parents think. Not knowing may be worse. In some ways, it's almost better to give too much information, so the healthy kid isn't left filling in the gaps, which is worse, or getting the message, 'I guess I shouldn't think about this, so I will numb a part of myself.'"

Having Company Helps

Having more than one healthy sibling in a family eases the pressure, said Brown University's Dr. Lobato. "If there are three or four kids, and only one has the illness, the healthy siblings have an experience of a sibling relationship without illness." Also, more than one sibling isn't getting enough attention, so it becomes less personal. From a practical point of view, she said, "If there are extra chores or responsibilities, they're spread among a couple of kids instead of just one."

On the other hand, Dr. Lewis said, when there are two healthy siblings, they may be split regarding the way they respond to the situation. "One may become overly solicitous, and the other may become withdrawn, indicating she can't be as good as the solicitous sibling," she said.

When More Than One Sibling Has IBD

As was pointed out in Chapter Two, the risk of IBD for someone who has a sibling with IBD is 30 times higher than for people in the general population, although it's rare for every sibling to have exactly the same degree of illness.

In some cases, a sibling with a less serious illness may assume the role of the healthy one. One such sibling is Rebecca, who has a largely non-symptomatic case of Crohn's that is limited to mouth sores and ulcers in her small intestine that don't bother her. Rather than empathizing with her younger sister, Hannah, who has a much more serious case, Rebecca carried on a contentious relationship.

"When I was diagnosed with Crohn's, I felt like I was stealing her disease," Rebecca said. "Everyone minimized my disease because I wasn't as sick. I always resented that." Rebecca kept a diary when Hannah was sick. "I'm kind of an attention seeker. When my parents were busy taking care of Hannah, I said I felt shocked at how they were ignoring me. I'd tell my mother that she thought I was fat, that she liked Hannah more, that I *knew* she liked her more, and that she's more special than I am. I was kind of maniacal. I went out of my way to make things hard for her. It makes me sad to think about," said Rebecca, who is now in her mid-20s.

For her part, Hannah, still chronically ill and struggling, strained to understand why her sister, who was in total remission, would react so negatively to her own Crohn's. "She gets scared when she sees the picture of her colon and comes back crying," Hannah said, somewhat derisively. "I don't understand, because a remission is a remission. It bothers me sometimes."

Clearly, Rebecca and Hannah are temperamentally different. "I couldn't in a million years understand how it's been for her," Rebecca said. "Hannah's a silent sufferer. I've always admired her strength. She wanted to spare everyone the burden of her suffering. That's admirable, but she could have cried on my shoulder. She never did that."

Rebecca thinks that when Hannah chose a summer job writing obituaries for people in hospice, she was working out her own grief about her Crohn's disease. "She told me she was crying in her cubicle, because she thought of herself in that situation. I don't think I could do that. Not at all."

Relationships That Work

On the other hand, sometimes the chemistry between siblings works well. Lauren, 17, was diagnosed with ulcerative colitis, leaving her sister, Carly, 14, to take care of herself. Carly didn't mind. "She's always been a low maintenance kind of kid," her mother, Tracy, said.

Lauren and Carly's situation is interesting, because, according to Dr. Lobato, younger siblings are usually not expected to take care of older siblings. Yet, Carly was astute about her family's situation and thoughtful about how her own behavior affected them. "I lay low and try not to cause any problems," she told me. "It's a lot of stress on my parents, so I try not to create a lot of drama and keep them calm. I've gotten used to not having as much attention because of all her doctor's appointments and everything. I'm kind of accustomed to being more independent, because she needs more attention. She's had anxiety issues, and I'm glad she has the attention to help her. If I have something going on, I can still talk to my parents. It's not like I'm left behind. After a while, I've gotten used to it."

Carly recognized that stress triggered her sister's symptoms, another reason she strived to keep stress levels low. "We used to fight a good amount over TV," she said. "I can't really do that because I can't get her stressed out. It's hard to try to get over it and not get mad. It's hard to keep it bottled up, but if it makes her feel better, it's fine. My parents have talked it over with me and told me that if we want to help her get better, we have to keep the stress down."

With her sister about to leave home for college, Carly imagined the house would be a lot quieter, but not necessarily less challenging. "I don't know if it'll be more stressful knowing she's on her own or less stressful because they'll have less to worry about," she said of her parents. She was sure of one thing, though. "It'll be less stress for me, because I'll have more time in the bathroom. I won't have to wait for her to get out of there in the morning."

Carly may encounter another unexpected challenge, according to Dr. Kodman-Jones. "When things calm down, healthy siblings don't know how to open back up and really talk about what's going on with them, because they're used to being more independent," the psychologist said. "When the sick child gets better or goes away from home, the self-sufficient sibling may resent having their independence whittled away as parents begin to pay more attention to them."

Forging a Life's Work from the Sibling Relationship

Keren was three years older than her brother Gideon, who died of complications from Crohn's at age 26. She became a psychotherapist after years of watching and intervening in her brother's illness. She had been aware of their parents' focus on him and of all the trips to the doctor. Gideon was diagnosed when she was 12, so Keren was old enough to be left alone when her mother was at the hospital for Gideon's many surgeries.

"I was left by myself or with my dad," she recalled. "I'm definitely sensitive to children being forgotten or overlooked. I think that was probably hard for me, but I wasn't a kid that demanded a lot of attention. He was the kind of kid who would have liked to be the center of attention. It was our natural temperaments. It affected me, and I wasn't quite sure as a kid how to resolve that." Keren's doctoral thesis focused on the relationship between healthy siblings and siblings suffering with medical illness.

Caring for a Sibling with IBD

Not every culture regards individuality highly, observed Dr. Lobato. In some places, she said, siblings don't necessarily compete for equal amounts of attention and material things. Western culture is "very individualistic and believes that every child has a right to his or her own trajectory. Now, think of a different culture," she said. "Go to South America, where there are many children in a family and the primary connection is between siblings. You're expected to take care of your brother and sister. If a kid in that culture has an illness that takes more time and attention, it takes away from everybody and nobody blinks an eye. It's your role to take care of anybody younger than you. Latino families have a collective orientation that says, 'I'm not as important as my whole family.' "

This is true in other non-Western cultures as well. Caring, patience, and loyalty characterized Nandita's care for her younger sister, Suri, who was diagnosed with ulcerative colitis at 20. After her diagnosis, Suri, an engineering student in India, returned home to Nepal. They had lost their mother when Suri was 9, so Nandita, 23, stayed home to care for her. "I just didn't show her my sadness," Nandita told me. "I just tried to say, 'This is going to work out. People are in much worse situations.' She always feared not having anyone around to help her when she needed them," Nandita added. "She has this fear of being alone. With ulcerative colitis, she gets really weak. Just being with her, spending time with her, being there in her presence made her comfortable. She was very lonely. She missed being outside, missed her college, her friends. She missed out on everything."

Suri noted that Nandita was her caretaker, but that she left home after she married and she wasn't around when Suri was bedridden with colitis. Suri said this not to blame her sister, but to emphasize her own isolation and fear. Soon after her sister left, Suri met a man online. She is now married with a young son.

A Young Child's Misunderstanding

Age seems not to correlate with siblings' maturity regarding chronic illness. Some younger siblings are considerate of their brother or sister with IBD, and some older ones show resentment about ceding attention to their ill brother or sister. It all comes down to temperament.

"I think it was hard at times for her," LeAnne said about her daughter, Trista, who is a year younger than her sister, Trinity. Trinity was hospitalized with ulcerative colitis when she was 8 years old. "When Trinity passed a lot of blood, Trista knew that going to the hospital didn't mean a day or two. It meant weeks at a time when she wanted me and I was at the hospital. We were very lucky to have my in-laws and friends who would take care of Trista. She kind of got rotated throughout the family — her uncle and aunt one night and grandma the next night. My husband would come home from work and spend two, three hours with her, and then he'd go to bed because he has to get up 4:30 or 5 in the morning."

One afternoon, when Trinity came home from the hospital after a grueling period of illness, Trista treated her with great love and affection. That night, LeAnne woke up and panicked because she couldn't find Trista anywhere. "She wasn't in her bed or anywhere I looked. Just as I turned the corner, I realized she was in bed with Trinity, holding her. In the morning, I told her, 'I don't want you lying with Trinity because I'm afraid you might hurt her if you bump her stomach.' Trista replied, 'I'm sorry, Mommy, but I thought the angels were going to take her during the night and I lay down so I could go with her to heaven.' She thought her sister was going to die," LeAnne said. "It scared her. It was hard on her. She couldn't fully understand everything that was going on."

Conclusion

In addition to advising parents to be as frank as possible with healthy siblings about what's going on with the sick one, Dr. Lewis advises parents to be open to having their healthy kids feel whatever they feel, including the feeling that it's not fair.

She suggests that parents give their healthy children a journal and encourage them to write in it, telling them, for example: "'Maybe I'm caught up in a crisis, but as soon as it's over, I'll read your journal.'" This way, parents can convey how important it is for them to understand how their healthy children feel about what's going on in the household. Parents can also tell their healthy children, "'If you can't tell me at this moment, you can tell me on paper and we'll come back and talk about it,'" said Dr. Lewis. "Any way a parent can hold rapport with a kid to express their range of feelings is important."

CHAPTER SIXTEEN
Working with IBD

Congratulations. You've run the gauntlet. You've made it through elementary school, high school, college, and perhaps even graduate school, managing your Crohn's disease or ulcerative colitis. Now, you're at the beginning of your career or in the market for a job, and IBD still follows you wherever you go. Even if you are not symptomatic, in the back of your mind you may have some insecurity about whether your disease will unexpectedly show up to interfere with your goals. And if you are symptomatic, you wonder whether to inform your employer. If you decide not to, you strategize about how to hide your disease, and that is inevitably stressful.

Many jobs that normally carry stress place an even heavier burden on people with IBD. David, who works with health-care organizations as a consultant, said that job stress probably contributes to his getting cramps, "and I'm a person built on stress." If he needs an emergency Crohn's appointment, he's often in a hospital where he can get one on site. He reserves his doctor's appointments for Fridays, when he has a little more flexibility. "No matter what job I chose, I'd find a way to keep myself stressed," David said. "I thrive off of it."

How people with IBD cope with stress obviously varies. When stress levels get too high to manage, some people change jobs. Some change careers. Some stick with whatever they're doing and take on more responsibility. What people with Crohn's and ulcerative colitis share is that stress usually affects their physical health. And worrying about their job stress makes it worse. What follows are some examples of how people with IBD manage their working lives, as well as examples of the range of attitudes they have toward their work.

Managing Stress

People with IBD whom I interviewed tended, curiously, to be attracted to high-stress work. At the very least, people with IBD treated their jobs as if they were high stress.

James was cold-calling people, working 14 hours a day, and studying to pass his licensing exams to become a financial adviser. He was also throwing up in the shower and feeling "really stressed out," which was not helping his severe ulcerative colitis. When we spoke, he was working as a financial analyst for hedge funds. "Now it's not too bad," he said. "It could be a stressful job, but I don't work long hours." When James found out that the global head of his group had had his colon removed at age 14 because of ulcerative colitis, he felt immensely comforted. "He was finishing my sentences for me," James said gratefully. "If I ever needed surgery, he'd know why I was out. That was a relief."

Although teaching is not usually considered a particularly physical line of work, it can be challenging for those with IBD who teach young children. Rose was student-teaching third graders, who sit at low desks, which required her to bend over to help them, thus putting pressure on her large intestines. Her ulcerative colitis flared so badly she barely got through the semester. "I was so inflamed," she said, "every move I made felt like my colon was tearing."

Rose said that her master teacher would tell her about her IBS, "as if it were the same thing and she kept talking on and on and on and then asked me to carry heavy stuff around. It was shocking. I thought she'd be more understanding." After getting her degree, Rose got a job in teaching but decided not to tell her principal or the school's office of human resources about her colitis. "There isn't a day when I don't think about it," she said. "Even when I don't have any symptoms, it's always in the back of my mind. Everything I do is to keep my colitis at bay."

Rachel understood the effect her job as a newspaper reporter was having on her Crohn's disease. "I just threw myself into it. I just worked and worked until I was completely exhausted," she said. "I had some really terrible times, because I do a lot of court reporting and court will not stop for you to go to the toilet. I had a lot of near misses with that. I basically just became determined that my illness wouldn't stop me."

Fortunately for Rachel, her newspaper had compassionate editors. "We have very few staff and a lot of pressure," she said. "My being away from work now is a nightmare for me, but they've been great. They tell me, 'You shouldn't have to be an iron woman. You don't have to prove your illness doesn't control you.' My boss forced me to take time off. I feel that I'm very lucky to work for such understanding people."

When we spoke, Rachel had been off from work for more than 14 weeks, including a week in the hospital for an emergency operation to remove her large intestine and create a colostomy. "In the industry I work in," she said, "no matter how I tried not to let it, the illness held me back. Other people will get projects I should get and promotions I should get. I'm a bit of a workaholic. I worry that I will look back and think that if I didn't have colitis, I could have achieved so much more in my life." She later left to work at a larger, and presumably more stressful, newspaper.

April's challenge in her first year of teaching was how to follow the rules about not running in the hallways, even when she needed to get to a toilet quickly. Diagnosed with ulcerative colitis at age 26, she said, "You have students you just can't leave. When I could, I would walk as quickly as I could to get to a bathroom, because you're not supposed to run. It got to the point that when I finally got to a restroom, I didn't care anymore about how it sounded. I wouldn't even flush while I was going, to mask the noise I make. I seriously thought I might go on disability."

Changing Jobs

Leaving a job because it makes you sick is certainly a way to take care of yourself. The question is whether your next job will be an improvement or something that creates the same problems you had before. The answer lies in luck and in your personality. Are you drawn to high stress jobs that you just can't help taking on? Or do you resolve to change your life and health for the better even if it disrupts your work life?

Lucy worked as a teacher right out of college, and she soon recognized that she couldn't take the stress. "When I get nervous, I always get an inflammatory bowel reaction," she said. However, she jumped from the frying pan into the fire when she graduated from law school and took a job with a large New York City law firm. The pressure, not surprisingly, proved too great and she moved with her husband back to her hometown and clerked for a judge for a year, a job she loved. She then joined a small litigation law firm where she has enjoyed a reduced stress level and a healthier gut. She attributes this to having "more experience, feeling more comfortable as a lawyer and having a clerkship under my belt," she said. "Philadelphia is less stressful than New York, the people are nicer and it's a smaller firm with less financial pressure." At the time I interviewed her, Lucy was pregnant, and she intended to work full time after the baby was born.

Shawn's Crohn's disease had gone haywire the previous year, when he was employed as a production coordinator for a visual effects company. "I was working 60-hour weeks for six months," he said. "It was during that job that I got sick. I'd only been in the industry for a year. I worried about everything."

He switched to a job with Industrial Light & Magic, the company that moviemaker George Lucas founded when he was making the original "Star Wars" movie. "The company I'm at now seems quite understanding," said Shawn, whose Crohn's disease was more under control. "The more I do my job, the more experienced I am and the less stressful it becomes." And the less stress he shoulders, the better he feels. "I've started to learn the things I need to worry about and what's not a big deal," he said. "If you make an error, you can fix it. The show will still go on. It won't be the end of the world. You don't have to stress about it."

Getting to Work

Commuting, a necessary part of the work day, can be a nightmare for people with IBD. There is no bathroom on most local trains or along freeways and stress about this can build until it feels as though your intestines will burst.

Maureen took the Metro every day from her suburban Maryland home to her first job as a financial analyst for a telecommunications company, but she couldn't get to downtown D.C. without stopping and getting off four or five times to go to the bathroom. "The medications weren't holding it together anymore," she said. "I'd get to the office and sleep at work because I couldn't stay awake." However, she added, "My boss was wonderful and helped me as much as she could. Then it progressed to where I couldn't travel. I couldn't function." Maureen was laid off just as she was readying herself for surgery to remove her colon, which was fine with her.

Maureen's doctors told her to look into careers that were low stress and, initially, she followed the directive. "Funny thing is, when I finished my surgery, I was working at a hair salon as a receptionist. Then I moved into trade shows, where, professionally, my stress levels are off the charts. That's how it's always been. I try very hard to stay calm, but I'm not."

Sherry, who has ulcerative colitis, took a job in the city right after finishing college, and she remembers days when she would get off the train several times during the 10-mile trip to go to the bathroom. At one point, she called her mother in hysterics from a station asking to get picked up and brought home, because she couldn't make it all the way to work. She thought, "I can't live like this the rest of my life."

Sherry has adjusted with the help of Remicade, which has quieted her symptoms. "The second I wake up, I'll go to the bathroom. I can usually finish before I go to work and I'm fine for the rest of the day." She doesn't go to the bathroom at work unless she can't hold it, because of her self-consciousness about the noises she makes. "I'll flush when

I'm going," she added. "I still get nervous about the sounds."

The Pros and Cons of Openness

People with IBD sometimes fear that their job security might be at stake if they talk about their Crohn's disease or ulcerative colitis to their employers or co-workers. But this carries its own price. Hiding makes it difficult to feel comfortable in your own skin. And yet, until something happens to force the issue, many people prefer not to talk about the discomfort they're in all day. That was the way I handled my years in daily journalism, until I needed to take time off to recuperate from the fatigue and blood loss from a particularly bad flare. My job wasn't at risk at all and I returned to it. Ultimately, I decided to quit because I didn't feel I would get better as long as I maintained an unhealthy routine of working on deadline. As I had grown older, work that had once been a joy had turned sour.

Colin, who worked for a small-town newspaper in Ohio, told me he kept his colitis secret for a long time "You can't say, 'I have to go,' he explained. "I felt my editors wouldn't understand. I didn't tell them until it was becoming clear I had to have surgery and needed time off." As it turned out, Colin's bosses understood his situation and he still works at the newspaper. Nevertheless, Colin expressed pride about the silence he had maintained for years. "Not that I was embarrassed by my colitis," he said. "I didn't want people to think differently about me, to think that I was diseased. I didn't want them to pity me. I never missed a day when I was sick, never missed an event, never took a sick day, even though I should have."

Joshua, a former chaplaincy intern in the Midwest, told me that chaplains are taught "about the spiritual need for self-care, but we were really expected to push ourselves despite physical illness. I was doing five overnights or on-call shifts a month, which meant being at the hospital. So I had a lot of sleep deprivation." Joshua had a flare-up of his Crohn's disease during his internship. "I was completely exhausted. I was taking Flagyl and Cipro and steroids at one point."

Being open about his Crohn's was a mixed blessing. Joshua found that his pastoral care became more relevant when he revealed to patients that he had Crohn's. "I was able to be more empathic and compassionate because of how I could relate, because I had done so much work thinking about these sorts of questions, about how it affects my life," he said. "And yet, I felt the need to cover. There was some shame." He was also afraid of having his position jeopardized if his disease became active, Joshua added, which would mean he'd need to take time off from work. His concerns had some basis. He knew someone without IBD who'd been fired because she had taken time off for illness.

When Joshua was working as a rabbi in a synagogue, the decision about whether to keep his Crohn's confidential was even more challenging. "I'd be quicker to talk about my father's suicide than my Crohn's," he told me. "I'm worried about the implications for my job. If I have a chronic illness, I'm concerned that the synagogue board will look at me differently and think of it as a liability. It's not easy to talk about suicide, but it's a historical moment in my past. I have a pulpit from which to speak to the community without an intermediary; once my Crohn's is out there, I don't control the narrative."

214

Getting Laid Off

Let's presume that you're working hard to cope with your IBD and you do the best work you can at your job. So, if you are laid off and you suspect it happened because of IBD, the resentment and despondency you feel can be exponentially worse.

Louie worked for a small pharmaceutical company for 14 years. The company was sold, and although Louie said he had an excellent track record and was head of his department, he had taken so many sick days for his Crohn's disease that they told him his job had been eliminated. "I think they did it because I have too many health issues," he said. "So when it came down to who they were going to keep, they didn't want to keep the sick guy. To me it was a big loss, not just for my daughter and myself, but also for the fact that my job was my baby. I hired every single person in my department, including my own boss. That was difficult." When we spoke, Louie was at home, living on federal disability benefits.

LoriAnn, who was diagnosed with ulcerative colitis at 21, had been working since she was 15, and she took two jobs while still in high school. "I had a really good work ethic," she said. "When I turned 18, I went straight to the corporate world, moved from packing and shipping into inventory, and when I got sick, I couldn't work anymore and got fired. I went from being able to work to not being able to work, because I had to go to doctors." LoriAnn tried taking waitressing jobs but she was fired because she couldn't work for a couple of days due to illness.

When we spoke, LoriAnn was again working two jobs, one during the week at a software company and the other during weekends as a hostess in a restaurant at a Disney resort. "I'm hoping I don't have a problem with this job," she said. "I haven't met my manager yet. I'm going to have to tell him about my colitis. If I have to go to the bathroom, would they rather have me go to the bathroom for five minutes or send me home the rest of the day?"

Finding Meaning in Work

Anyone, sick or not, may stay in a job they've lost interest in because they can't afford to lose their health insurance. In a fluid job market, however, the opportunity to create a better work life is tempting, particularly when your IBD is affected by too much stress. You may even begin to ask yourself existential questions, including whether your work could benefit your life or society at large and even whether you should be involved with IBD and its treatments. Several people I interviewed worked at IBD organizations, because they knew their employers would understand their illness. Some struck out on their own as entrepreneurs, seeking to make a living helping others with IBD.

Joel, who has ulcerative colitis, felt handcuffed to his job as lead engineer on a multimillion-dollar government program. "It was interesting, when you're dealing with the FBI," he said. "It's cool and fun, but I wasn't tapped into what my mission on this earth was." He moved to another company on the sales side, where he made more money and could work from home, which was convenient because he had easy access to his own bathroom and he could lie down in his bedroom when he felt fatigued.

When we spoke, he'd left that job to become a health coach. "As I go through being a yoga teacher and take other types of courses and workshops, I realize you have to educate yourself on how to deal with stress and stressful situations."

Joel found that even working in a New-Agey field such as health coaching caused stress to affect his gut. He went to Toastmasters, an organization that strengthens one's public speaking skills. "Before I'd go in front of the room, I'd have to go to the bathroom," he said. Joel's stress travels straight to his stomach.

Shira also has transformed her ulcerative colitis into a career, which began when she feared that she might develop colon cancer one day. She teaches yoga, eats with great discipline and coaches others in her situation to do the same. "I've created an online program," she said. "The program is basically what I've done for myself. It includes diet, cleansing, yoga, and meditation. I've gotten some good reviews. And I feel that I've been able to help some people. I've embraced colitis and taken it on full force. I've taken action, not let it take its course. I've coached clients around it. I've created a life around it. I've written a book that's on Amazon."

When Work Just Works

Many people working with IBD have had positive experiences with their employers and co-workers. They find compassion and collegiality where others experience difficulties.

Adina, who has ulcerative colitis, works as a fundraiser for a major organization. Her job is "demanding but flexible," she said. "I'm either meeting people or on the phones, so if I can't physically come to the office it's okay. I'm very honest with my supervisor if I need to go home or go to a doctor's appointment. We just had a 1,000-person gala, and I was working around the clock. If I work late, I try to go in late."

Alyssa, who was an assistant to the director of student housing at San Diego State University, said that while it's "definitely a stressful job, I've been very open with my boss about having Crohn's disease. His wife has multiple sclerosis, so he understands. I exercise, so I can get all the life stresses out and be able to relax. At the end of the day, when it's my time to leave, I leave. I know I can't hold onto that stress the way I always have. Any time I have any sort of stress, I have a hard time eating. Stress and Crohn's are completely related for me."

Ben handles the stress of being a standup comedian with Crohn's by emotionally detaching himself from any pain he may be having. "I have never have missed a gig," he told me. "I'm really good at acknowledging that I'm in pain and then forgetting about it. I've done plenty of gigs where I've felt kind of awful, but I can keep my sphincters shut enough that I know I won't have an accident in front of other people. When I'm onstage, I'm not a party to the rules of how I'm feeling. A hundred percent of what I do is feeling the experience the audience is having."

Conclusion

The most prominent theme that emerged from these interviews was that high-stress jobs inflamed IBD. And yet, these were precisely the jobs that drew IBD patients, like moths to a flame. The challenge is to support yourself financially without breaking down physically.

In this book's introduction, I mentioned a cheerleading message — "Yes, it's hard, but you can do it!" — and I concluded that it didn't scratch the surface of the complexities of living with IBD. But Chelsea, a musical theater actress with Crohn's disease, lives up to that motto. And even though most of us don't have the grit (or talent) to star in a Broadway musical, her story may be helpful to those who are prone to giving up.

Diagnosed at age 13, Chelsea attended the Boston Conservatory, a top school for musical theater. From there, she was cast in the Broadway production of "The Little Mermaid" as Ariel's sister, Andrina, and as the understudy for Ariel. After about a year and a half, the actress playing Ariel was hired to do another show and the company did a nationwide search for the next Ariel. Chelsea was hired to play the role until the show closed.

Throughout her career, Chelsea's physical stamina has been supported by regular doses of Remicade, which she dutifully takes wherever she is performing and which keeps any flares at bay. But her medication-induced vulnerable immune system plagues her. "I feel like I'm constantly dealing with different medical things that aren't directly related to Crohn's, but because my immune system is lower, I deal with new little things," she said. "For example, a year ago I had these swollen, bleeding gums that came out of nowhere. And I have really good teeth."

Chelsea volunteered at Mount Sinai Hospital in New York City, counseling young people with IBD. "Please don't give up!" she wrote in a hospital newsletter. "Don't ever say, 'I can't,' because you can. Just to live with Crohn's or colitis makes you stronger. If we understand what we have to deal with, but take action to find the right medicine and right diet, we can move forward. It is always a battle, but I believe that the real fight sometimes is finding the power to think positively and in continuing to strive for your dreams!"

While that sounds a little, well, Disney-like, and doesn't apply to everyone who is struggling with runaway symptoms, there is a large grain of truth in her words. While a positive attitude and the right diet will hardly enable you to work at a high-stress job, the mind-gut connection is an unavoidable feature of coping with IBD in the workplace or outside it. People feel a boost every time they discover a sports figure or another public figure with Crohn's disease or ulcerative colitis, because it means that person wasn't held back from achieving challenging life goals. It's a lesson everyone with IBD can take in.

CHAPTER SEVENTEEN

Talking and Support

"Suffering — whether physical, emotional, spiritual, or as often the case, all three —can be a doorway to transformation.... We all have within us access to a greater wisdom, and we may not even know that until we speak."

— Dean Ornish, M.D., president and director of the Preventive Medicine Research Institute

As a teenager and young woman, I made my life immeasurably more difficult because I remained silent about my ulcerative colitis, which, had I been honest about it, was the main fact of my life at the time. I felt intense loneliness and stress while trying to act as if I were healthy. I usually hid the fact that I desperately needed to get to a bathroom. I silently suffered through such severe cramps that the pains of childbirth later felt like an anti-climax. I met no one else who talked openly about having IBD, so I felt completely alone in my struggles.

As it turns out, I was not alone in trying to create a mask of normalcy in order to face the world. Most people I spoke with had similar reasons for silence: They were self-conscious and afraid to be judged, pitied, teased, or regarded as frail. Many patients didn't know how to talk about their IBD, in part because they couldn't find the right words and in part because they feared that people would not know how to respond.

Heathir, the mother of two children with Crohn's disease whom I referred to previously, summed up the issue bluntly. "Crohn's is an icky disease," she said. "Nobody wants to talk about it. That's why it doesn't get all the press, like cancer or even rheumatoid arthritis and other autoimmune diseases do. It's not cool to talk about going to the bathroom 15 times a day where you have diarrhea and throw up. You don't see anyone walking about with an 'I Got Guts' wristband, because nobody wants to talk about it."

When I was growing up with IBD, there were no advocates to turn to, nobody to talk to except my doctor and my parents. Today, you would think that the proliferation of websites, Facebook pages, summer camps, and CCFA support groups would mean that patients would feel less alone. Many do, but not everyone. Most of the young people I spoke with went through a stage when they could not openly talk with peers about their IBD. Most changed their ways later on and were happier for it. By virtue of the fact that they spoke with me, everyone I interviewed had decided to open up, although in one interview that began in a coffee shop, the person mumbled softly, looked around furtively to make sure no one could hear what he was saying, and then decided he preferred to conduct the interview in the privacy of his home.

Coming Out of Hiding

The sense of shame and inhibition that keeps families and patients from openly discussing IBD creates added anguish that can last for years.

"When I got Crohn's disease at 13, my parents told me not to tell anyone," said Jerry, a 33-year-old writer in New York City. "I told one person in the next six years. I'd be taking all these pills and hiding them from people. During meals at a friend's house, I'd hide the pills under the table before I put them in my mouth and swallowed, because I was so ashamed of taking them."

After we spoke, Jerry called his mother and asked her why she had ordered his silence. "She said people would treat me like an invalid," he reported back, "and that this was our problem as a family, not anyone else's."

When I later spoke with Jerry's mother, Deborah, she affirmed his account. It turned out that she also had Crohn's disease and she had taken Prednisone for it for a decade. "The culture in our family is to say nothing," she said. "We didn't tell anyone. I'm sure that did him no favors." Deborah asked Jerry about how her insistence on his silence had affected him. She said Jerry told her he felt as if it were his fault that he had the disease and that he should be embarrassed. "We just didn't want him treated differently," she said in a matter-of-fact tone, without remorse.

Experiencing social isolation while struggling through IBD is clearly not good for your health. Nevertheless, many people with IBD suffer symptoms in silence for at least a period of their illness until they learn how much better it is to have company in their misery.

Marisa lived with her parents into young adulthood while being incapacitated by ulcerative colitis, and in her isolation she came to understand that seclusion was not serving her well. She realized that she needed peers in her life who would understand what she was going through. She explored the Internet and came across an IBD blog and YouTube videos featuring people who were boldly out of their shell. She also discovered a Facebook page called "The Great Bowel Movement" and started chatting online with one of the page's founders. They bonded over their mutual sadness at having loved and lost their ability to compete in high school sports. Inspired by her Internet interactions, Marisa decided to emerge from her silence and write her own blog, describing her journey from her first symptoms to the aftermath of surgery and beyond. Her intention was to let others know they were not alone. She blogged under the titles "Keeping Things Inside is Bad for My Health" and "Journaling IBD."

But not everyone chooses to be so open about IBD. Some of the people I interviewed indicated that they didn't want to talk with friends about IBD at all. When Kevin was diagnosed in high school, his resolution to remain silent left him lonely and depressed and permitted rumors to spread. In high school, some classmates speculated that he had AIDS. Consumed with stress, he became suicidal.

So, when Kevin was hospitalized, he decided not to allow any visitors. "I need to be alone to get myself together and rest," he told me. "I like to be at peace. I don't want to be questioned about it. I don't want people lecturing me about what I need to do." Kevin, who grew up in Louisiana, believed in voodoo, which holds that if you talk about something, it will act up. It so happened that Louisa, a young Jewish woman with Crohn's disease, described the same belief. She said her family worried that talking about her Crohn's would give energy to it and thereby cause it to flare. She called this superstition a Jewish thing. Kevin considered it a Louisiana thing. Perhaps it's a human thing.

The fear of judgment is another motivator for keeping silent. Chava speaks cautiously about her ulcerative colitis and only on an as-needed basis. She has to be fairly certain that her listener will empathize rather than criticize. The first time she spoke with someone outside her family was two years after her diagnosis, when she was 20. A colleague mentioned she had had a fissure that made her constipated. "I tested the waters," Chava said. "When you see the other person is not disgusted, you feel more comfortable." She started by responding, "'Yeah, I have problems in the bathroom.'" You move on to uncontrollable diarrhea," she said, "and then you move on to 'Sometimes, I can't make it to the bathroom.'"

Even after that conversation, Chava remained guarded. Only when silence became unwieldy did she disclose to her running partner that she was sick. "I couldn't always make it to her house on time because I was trying to go to the bathroom before I left my house," she said. "Sometimes, I'd say, 'We have to stop running.'" She finally allowed herself to be vulnerable and she told her friend, "I have to get back to the bathroom."

Worrying about how others will react if you openly discuss your IBD can create anxiety and social paralysis. Internalized fears begin to feel like reality. Colin was diagnosed at 22 with ulcerative colitis and he journeyed through his illness largely alone for the next six years. "My friends, God bless them, don't understand what it's like to have the disease," he said. Colin worried about how his friends would react if he told them about his colitis. He was so self-protective that his close friends didn't even know he was sick until he was hospitalized for surgery.

None of his imagined outcomes for speaking up were positive. "Even if they didn't have a reaction when they hear you have a disease that involves body waste, I wondered whether they would think it's gross, wouldn't understand, or worse, would find it funny. My friends and I always poked fun at each other. The people who are the meanest to you are your friends, they say," he said, ruefully. "I didn't know if I could get the emotional support I needed."

Then, Colin's life turned around for the better after his colon was removed and replaced with a J-pouch. After his surgery, he decided to open up. He became connected to the CCFA, shared his story in a group setting, and formed a circle of friends who would understand what he'd been through.

When you're a teenager, social pressures can lead you down some pretty dubious roads, but when you have IBD, those roads can be especially treacherous. Thomas wouldn't talk to his friends about his Crohn's and, while in high school, he went to the mountains to spend the weekend with them. They were drinking Jack Daniels. He joined them and ended up in the emergency room. "You want to be one of the guys?" his mother, Laura, told him in a fury. "You're putting them in the position that you could have died on them. How would they have known? They're not your friends if you can't tell them what you've got." He's been very open since.

Getting Help

Simone Leo never felt any reluctance to speak about her Crohn's / colitis, which was diagnosed when she was 19. She found comfort in support groups. "It's such a value to feel connected to people who have the same feelings and thoughts you have," she said as she sat in a meeting hall at Camp Oasis, where she was a resident social worker working with kids with IBD. "You feel validated. You're not alone. You're part of a bigger whole. I've helped people get control of their illness and helped them learn how to communicate with their doctors." She plainly felt as helped as the ones she helped.

When Jonathan was diagnosed with Crohn's disease at 22, he was convinced that he could do anything he set his mind to do. But when he tried to enroll in the Israel Defense Forces and had to tell them about his Crohn's, he was rejected on the spot. "Saying I had Crohn's had very real consequences. It said to me, be careful about this information, because people will assume you can't do things," he said. "The last thing I wanted to do was talk to someone who's writing a book about Crohn's and colitis and tell them about my experience," he confessed. "But it's healing just talking about it."

Jonathan read stories in CCFA newsletters and realized that he didn't have IBD as badly as people who were unable to leave their homes or who were worried that they would have an accident in the mall. "I've experienced just enough of it to relate and be grateful it's not my situation," he said. "I've had diarrhea, but not every day of my life. So, hearing other people's stories and telling my own story provides a lot of comfort and support." Jonathan believes that opening up about his Crohn's has contributed to his improved health. "I've come to terms with reality and gotten my s—- out and not left it inside. And then the s—- can be used for fertilizer. It fertilizes so, so much. It brings healing and growth to my soul."

Dr. Philip Yucht, a New Jersey-based therapist who has Crohn's, believes this: "The only reason not to tell anybody is if there is something you need to achieve that you think you can't if you tell.

"Teenagers worry about what people are going to think about them," Yucht said. "Will they be rejected by their friends who will not want to be around them and make fun of them? It depends on the personality of the kid," he said.

"Some kids handle that really well. The more shy individual might not."

In fact, virtually all the patients I spoke with felt relieved after they spoke up. Most had positive experiences like Stacey, who told a few friends almost in passing, at the urging of her mother, a psychologist. Stacey's friends did not let her down. "They had a great reaction," she said. "They wanted to learn more about it. They asked about the symptoms. They always want to know how I am feeling. Through the course of my colitis, I've never come across anyone who's made fun of me. I joke about it myself. When someone has to go to the bathroom, I'll say, 'Welcome to my life.' So there's nothing anybody could say that I haven't already said or thought of. It lets people be a lot more light-hearted about it."

The decision to engage in a support group can move you toward self-acceptance. This is how it was for Emmett, who saw a poster advertising a Crohn's support group while in college. It was the first time he had ever participated in such a group. "They talked about diet, drugs, what worked, what didn't work, what are you like in relationships and how do you deal with your friends," he said. Emmett described himself as "pretty adamant about my situation. I have it. This is what I am. I live with this."

Using Humor to Diffuse Discomfort

Ben, diagnosed at 21, avoids using his Crohn's disease in his standup comedy routine. But he wrote a novel so raw and funny about having Crohn's, it almost hurts to read it. He explained that he chose to confront his Crohn's in a novel, where he didn't have to directly confront his readers' reactions. He has not yet devised a standup routine to discuss his Crohn's.

"It's kind of a tough subject to talk about," he said. "It's about as intimate as you can get. The audience might get disgusted. I'm surprised how easily disgusted they are in general." He gauges their receptivity by talking about his hemorrhoids. "People are offended," he said. "It's way more offensive to *have* a hemorrhoid than to *talk* about it," he added — something that could also be said of IBD. "But it's definitely something I want to do."

Another Ben, a comedian based in Los Angeles who was diagnosed at 17, turned his Crohn's disease into a career. He created a website called benmorrison.org, and he does a standup routine called "Pain in the Butt." He has been on the cover of *Crohn's Advocate* magazine and has served as a product spokesman for the odor-eliminating product, "You Go, Girl."

Nevertheless, Ben reserves his Crohn's material for audiences that are largely peopled by individuals with IBD. When he performs before general audiences, he limits himself to a brief bit about how "comedians are comedians because of tragedy, and mine just happens to be that I grew up with all these weird medical problems. And I do mention that I sh— myself.' If I get a nervous laugh, I'll say 'I sh— myself right now. I'm serious.' "

Ben refrains from speaking about his intestinal problems at length in front of general audiences, because he doesn't want to wear out their good will. "For the most part, I save the real shebang for people who are going through it" — particularly at fundraisers for IBD organizations, he said. For them, Ben thoroughly owns his disease. He doesn't hold back when making fun of himself and his gastroenterologists.

"Not only are you out of control with diarrhea, you can't eat food anymore and, in addition to feeling like you've become a toddler again, you also have to have [an endless line] of people you don't know journeying into your ass to tell you they still don't know. When you come down to it," he told me, "that's why I do what I do. That set of circumstances is so foreign to everyone and almost so tragic, you have to f—-ing laugh about this. If you don't take the head of foam off this situation by laughing at it, it's going to be the biggest pile of sad. And who needs that?"

Ben has little patience for self-pity. "A lot of the psychosocial victimization that life has put on you is something you've invented," he said. "This is how I end my show. Once you have a heart-to-heart with someone," he told me, "nine times out of ten they'll say, 'I have MS, or cystic fibrosis, or my mom is going through chemotherapy.' Everyone has something. Everyone. Everyone has his own pain in the butt. You're going to find that once you're open about your Crohn's or colitis, your friends will be amazing. They probably need you to listen to them as much as you need them to listen to you. You need to show them you own something that seems so un-ownable."

Getting Support Online

Learning to be open on the Internet can break open the emotional floodgates and create a sense of safety while you communicate what is really going on with you. This, in turn, can make you feel better about being more honest about your IBD with friends and acquaintances.

IBD websites and Facebook pages have served as a boon not only to people with no geographical access to support groups but also to those who would rather not reveal themselves in face-to-face encounters. In all areas of life, the Internet combines anonymity with connection. For many with IBD, the Internet is a gateway to information and openness.

Alisa is socially connected. She is married and close to her family of origin. But "as much as I love my husband and family, I feel a general frustration that no one really understands what I'm talking about," she said. Diagnosed at 22, Alisa wanted to find a common bond with other people with IBD and so she began searching the Internet. The stories she read were a revelation to her. "Oh my God, there's a whole community of people who have ulcerative colitis," she told me with surprise. She found herself almost addicted to reading about others who had the disease, but it took nearly a year more to summon the courage to tell her own story online. "I'm trying not to regret all the time I was silent," she said. "Instead, I just know this is the right time I'm supposed to be reaching out." She embarked on writing a blog called "Tiny Little Ulcers."

Shawn was motivated to go online the year before we spoke, after he developed fistulas and abscesses. Although he had spent many years with his disease, the setback made him feel similar to someone just diagnosed with Crohn's. "I was afraid. I was scared," he said. "It had never happened to me before. I discovered a Crohn's forum board online with different sections for people with abscesses and fistulas. I discovered there were people who had it much worse than me and it put it into perspective for me." Until that point, he said, he had been asking, 'Why me?' and hating his disease. He wouldn't be the first person to experience gratitude by understanding that many others have it worse.

Nerissa knew no one else with ulcerative colitis when she was diagnosed at 23. She lacked basic information about her disease until she went online and found out that the disease that she thought affected only the middle-aged, the elderly, and herself afflicts many people her age and younger.

Although she was reluctant to reach out to individuals online, Nerissa did begin talking with her friends. She learned to become open and honest about it and they, in turn, put her at ease. "Most people who know me well know I have ulcerative colitis, and although I don't tell everyone about it, I am happy to speak about it frankly," she said. "I can understand why people go online to get support from others, and that's absolutely fine, but it is so important to speak to your loved ones, as they are the ones who can really help you. For instance, if I'm with my sister and brother-in-law in town and my colitis flares up, they notice the symptoms instantly and know exactly what to do," she said. "It's that kind of support that makes me feel less stressed and more able to get on with my life. It's okay having a good doctor, but it's not going to help when you're not having a fun time, when you're young and you're making excuses not to go out and you're a recluse. I think it's important for young people to have some community, whether it's online or not."

Not Everyone Wants Support

However, not everyone takes comfort from the Internet or local support groups. Some find others' stories to be depressing rather than uplifting, neither validating nor instructive. Perhaps you fear that absorbing yourself with online interactions means that IBD will take over your life, even if your life is already overtaken by IBD.

Carolyn, the mother of a son with Crohn's, observed that people who are most visible online are still looking for answers, since those who feel fairly well usually do not spend their time with online support groups. "You see numerous negative stories online," she said. "It can be scary. The same thing can occur with support groups. If you don't have problems, you're busy with life" and are not drawn to groups where members are still suffering.

Melissa, 28, found that reading online stories discouraged her. Online chat groups turned her off. "Sometimes, it's better if I don't go on there," she said. "I want to be positive. I want to share and encourage other people. There has to be some balance. I didn't want to go online and have it be a big downer."

Shawn didn't want to be known as a "Crohnie," as people with Crohn's disease sometimes refer to themselves. After an abscess was drained and Remicade arrested most of his symptoms, Shawn wanted to feel like "a normal person again. I want to be positive about it. Sure, I have to get an infusion once every two months and I have to be sure not to eat stupid things, but I can do anything I put my mind to, if I want to." So Shawn stopped going to the online Crohn's forum board because he didn't want to be "constantly reminded of this thing I had. I didn't want to pretend I didn't have it. I just didn't want it to be something I constantly thought about."

While people up and down the age spectrum do attend support groups, I heard again and again how young people felt uncomfortable because they were among the few young ones in the pack. So, when young people with IBD want to join a support group, they may find few that are not populated with older adults. Heathir said her son wanted to find a support group after his diagnosis with Crohn's disease.

"It's all adults," she said. "There was no pediatric support group." One reason for the preponderance of older people at support groups is that adults are more willing to articulate their problems with IBD than are younger people, who may still be getting adjusted.

When Laura was 18, she attended a CCFA support group soon after she was diagnosed with ulcerative colitis, but she found it depressing to be among older people with her disease. She thought, "They're going to die soon," she said. "That means I'm going to die soon." She didn't go back. Instead, she turned to the Internet and met young people like herself. The Internet became her support group for several years and people she met there are still online friends. But impending J-pouch surgery drove her back to her local support group, where she met Bev, her "guardian angel," who accompanied her to the hospital to serve as her advocate. After the surgery, Laura became president of a patient-run support group out of gratitude for what had been done for her. "I felt compelled," she said. "Other people needed my help. I wanted to give back locally and I wanted to be a face of someone who was younger, so that other people my age would think to themselves that they're not alone, that they not feel the way I felt for four or five years, when I couldn't connect with anybody."

Rachel, who was diagnosed at 13, fervently advocates for communicating about IBD. She wished she had followed her own advice sooner, "so I wouldn't have felt so hurt and bullied by people who didn't understand," she said. "As a youngster, you're easily scared. Your body is going through changes anyway. You're not sure what's happening. You can't talk to your friends." Now in her mid-20s, Rachel encourages other young people to check out online support groups, "where you can talk to other people and realize you're not alone. Don't keep it to yourself," she said heatedly. "Seek out other people who have it. Don't let other people call you names or say you're anorexic or have an eating problem. Small people can't see past what you look like. Tell them what you've got so they can understand what you're going through."

Isolation

When I worked for the *Philadelphia Inquirer*, I awoke one night to shivering, spasms and shaking such as I had never had before. It was 3 a.m. Who could I call at that hour? I was single, and my friendships were more acquaintance-like, not so close that I felt comfortable rousing someone from bed in the middle of the night. I waited it out until morning, when I called an emergency-room physician, the husband of a college friend. He surmised that I'd had an abscess in my colon. I never had shaking like that again, so I did nothing about it. Many years later, when I interviewed Colin for this book, I learned that he had had the exact same experience.

Colin worked for an Ohio newspaper while he fought through ulcerative colitis, but he never told his bosses what he was going through. "I never had a whiny, woe-is-me attitude," he said, but he acknowledged the "demands of being a reporter, of being somewhere where you don't know where the facilities are. I went to bathrooms in pretty bad places," he said. "You know you have to report on something. You can't say, 'Sorry, I have to go.' "

One late night while he was covering an event, he needed to run to the bathroom. "The only thing that came out was blood," he said. "The toilet was full to the top with blood. I looked at it. I went into shock. I started shaking, shivering, shaking. I was by myself. I didn't have any friends to call on. I lived by myself. I managed to make it home. I couldn't stop shaking. I just had to ride it out until the morning. There was no one I could talk to, no one I could call. I never had it before or again."

Reasons to Choose Silence

There are legitimate reasons why some young people do not want to speak about their IBD to friends and why others do, according to psychologist Fran Martin, who ran a parent support group at the Children's Hospital of Philadelphia and whose daughter was diagnosed with Crohn's at age 13. "Some kids are more comfortable keeping it private; others want to share the truth," she said. "It's hard for children to find other children they can talk with. Who wants to talk about poop? That's really what having IBD is about.

"The medical people are not very attuned to the impact of this disease on children and parents," she continued. "They're just not very psychologically attuned and parents are desperate. It shakes up your life really profoundly."

Although Fran organized a support group for parents of children with IBD to discuss the impact on their families, few parents showed up. "Those who came," Martin said, "seemed to really experience the benefit of being able to talk about their experience." There are many reasons why the turnout was so light, she said. Parents live busy lives, especially with a sick child. Spending an hour talking with other parents about IBD's impact on your family may seem like a luxury — and an unnecessary one at that.

There are reasons why some children do not see the benefits of sharing. "For kids, keeping it secret is a way to maintain a sense of control over something over which they have very little control," Martin said. However, the benefits of preserving control diminish over the years, as children transition into being teenagers and young adults. "The toll of maintaining a secret as an adult is that while you maintain surface control, you get caught in a trap of isolation, and it's emotionally detrimental," she said. "We're social creatures who find comfort when we find even a small group with whom we can share our stories."

What *Not* to Say to Someone with IBD

One of the reasons IBD patients offered for not talking about their IBD is that they fear the response will make them feel worse. Given the stories above, what is the best way, if you don't have IBD, to interact with a friend or acquaintance who does? Here are suggestions from Crohn's & Colitis Australia. (Crohn's & Colitis Australia, 2015)

(www.crohnsandcolitis.com.au/11-things-say-some-one-ibd/)

Let's start with what *not* to say and then proceed to the best approaches.

1. **"You don't look sick."**

To someone suffering from IBD, it is a double blow not to be believed. "It is a lonely disease," said Colin, "because people can't see it on the outside of you. People said I looked great. I didn't feel great. At the time, I wouldn't tell them I felt terrible on the inside." People who are very ill with IBD often look like everyone else. Don't challenge their assertion that they are ill.

2. **"I know what you're going through"**

If an IBD patient is reaching out to talk to you about the details of the condition, including diarrhea and rectal bleeding, it is best not to respond with details about your own digestive problems — or any other illness, for that matter. One of the beliefs commonly held by people with IBD is that no one fully understands what they're going through. It's wise not to confirm that belief by saying that you do.

3. "You've lost weight! You look great!"

A person with IBD who has lost weight due to illness does not want to hear that weight loss is a good thing. Chava's personal trainer told her she looked great after she lost 30 pounds in one month. After 12 years of working with him, she revealed to him that she had ulcerative colitis and that was why she had lost the weight so quickly and drastically.

4. "Come on, try a bite!"

People with IBD know what foods upset them and they stay away from them. Don't make it harder by encouraging them to eat what they don't want to.

5. You're so lucky — you can eat anything and stay skinny"

In the midst of a flare-up of IBD, the body is largely incapable of absorbing nutrients. Someone who looks wonderful may be suffering from being seriously depleted nutritionally. While a few people with whom I spoke were grateful to be skinny because of their IBD, most were trying to hold onto their calories in order not to look skeletal.

6. "You must have a lot of stress in your life"

Many people believe that stress causes inflammatory bowel disease. There's absolutely no evidence of this, although stress can make symptoms worse for people who already have IBD. A rogue immune attack on the digestive tract, sometimes genetic, sometimes not, is the cause of IBD.

7. "You've really put on weight!"

Prednisone causes quick weight gain and distended cheeks, called "moon face" or "chipmunk cheeks." People taking Prednisone are likely to be self-conscious about their appearance. Better not to say anything. They will lose the weight as soon as they stop taking the steroid. (Come to think of it, better not to say this to *anyone*, whether they have IBD or not.)

8. Can't you wait for the next exit?"

When someone with IBD tells you they have to go, they mean immediately, if not sooner. An inflamed colon does not wait for the next exit. This response brings up painful memories for Adina, whose parents felt frustrated before her diagnosis, because they had to stop so often so she could go to the bathroom. "My parents used to say, 'You can wait. You're a big girl.' They had no idea it was my colitis."

9. "Is it OK for you to eat that?"

Asking someone with Crohn's or colitis whether they should eat something means that you don't trust them to look after themselves. Besides, there is no one healthy way to eat if you have IBD. "One thing I saw in the Crohn's and Colitis support group," observed Elan, "is that some people can drink beer and others can't. Some say they can only eat leafy greens; others get sick with even a single leaf of spinach. There's no one approach that fits everyone."

10. "Why are you so tired?"

Jill's friends and family tried to get her to do things she was not up to by saying, for example, "Oh, come on. You can't be that tired." She would answer, "If you lost as much blood as I do with each bowel movement, you'd be pretty wiped out too."

In short, "Don't baby the person, said David Eisikovits, a counselor who co-leads a support group for the Manhattan chapter of the CCFA. "Give the person space and, if they want to talk, let them talk. Sometimes we get smothered in pity and it makes people with IBD feel very self-conscious, helpless and low."

What to Say to Someone with IBD

The following list was posted on Facebook. It can be valuable for anyone who knows someone with IBD, but doesn't know how to be helpful without being intrusive.

1. "Is there anything I can do to help?"
   Even if we say no, the question means a lot to us.
2. "I'd love to make you breakfast/lunch/dinner. Is there something special you'd appreciate?"
   This is especially thoughtful for those of us on special diets.
3. "Would you like to go for a walk/drive/bicycle ride?"
   Getting away from it all for a bit is wonderful.
4. "Would you like a hug?"
   Can't get enough of them!
5. "I'm sorry for what you are going through. I can't imagine the struggles." Unless you've got it, you likely won't "get it," so acknowledging that is appreciated.
6. "Would you like to hear a great joke/funny story?"
   Laughter really *is* the best medicine.
7. "If you feel like talking, I've got time to just listen."
   Sometimes, we just need to vent without having suggestions for treatments, diets, and alternative therapies offered up.

8. "So, I was reading the other day about [name of illness here] and found this interesting..."
    Sometimes, we also appreciate genuine concern and an interest in our situation that's not patronizing.
9. "Would you like me to go to your appointment with you?"
    While some doctor's visits are routine, some aren't, and company can take the sting out of the trying visits.
10. "Want to go to the art gallery/beach/mall/book store/coffee shop today?" Knowing that our lives don't have to revolve around our illnesses is important.
11. "I was wondering if you'd like some company today?"
    Time is the greatest gift.

Conclusion

After listening to more than 100 patients talk about their attitudes toward being open about IBD, I can confidently say that, as a rule, it is far more beneficial to speak out than to stay silent. It is better to seek out others with the disease, whether online or in person, than it is to be isolated. As I write this, these points seem obvious, but many of us live with IBD in the opposite way. Our shame, our self-consciousness and our desire for privacy trump the need for connection. If talking about it with friends and extended family is too difficult for you, perhaps you can begin by talking to a psychotherapist with whom you can find a safe space to practice talking about your IBD.

Talking about it will not cure the disease, but it will help you to adapt to it. And isn't that the ideal way to live with IBD? It isn't curable. It won't go away. But there are ways to integrate the illness into your life so that you don't feel possessed and overwhelmed.

"I don't want to be defined by the disease, but it's definitely a part of who I am" said Nicole, 18. "I'm not ashamed of it and I'm not going to try and hide it at all."

CHAPTER EIGHTEEN
The Upsides of IBD

Considering how many stories in this book chronicle the struggles of daily life with IBD, it may seem improbable to take into account the upside of having Crohn's disease or ulcerative colitis — that is, to understand the ways in which IBD can contribute to a deeper and more fulfilled life. And yet, all but two of the more than 100 people I interviewed cited at least one way that their Crohn's or colitis had enhanced their lives, if only in hindsight. They recognized the truth that when something huge like IBD ruptures your life, you emerge a different person, often for the better.

What follows is a sampling of the advantages patients have accrued by coping with IBD. They are not prettifying the disease. They are not presenting a Disney version of life with Crohn's disease or ulcerative colitis. These people engage in a daily scrimmage with IBD or its aftereffects. But even people who have lost organs or parts of organs and who have taken strong medication with serious side effects have found practical benefits as they try to banish IBD to the sidelines of their lives.

Appreciation

Some patients discussed how much they appreciated being alive and having a disease whose severity wasn't life threatening. Dahlia initially said she saw no upside to having IBD, but then she went on to describe an important one. "I was very aware of the fragility of life at a fairly young age," she said. "I think that definitely came from my

Crohn's experience. You have to appreciate life. I don't approach it in a morbid way, but I've been aware of stories that aren't so good as mine."

Kenneth wants people to know that "if anyone has stomach issues, they never have to worry about it around me. I totally understand. You never have to be embarrassed. [Crohn's has] made me more sensitive as a manager to medical things that pop up," he said. "In the grand scheme of diseases, Crohn's is not horrible to have. I have a glimpse of people with more severe handicaps and disorders they have to deal with. I feel blessed."

Rachel, who was diagnosed with Crohn's/colitis at age 13, echoed almost every other patient when she said that she'd rather not have IBD. But, she added, "I can't imagine my life without it." She paused and thought some more. "The only good thing that's come out of it is that I've recently made some good friends," she said. "In the hospital, I made a friend who also has Crohn's who'll be a friend for life." Then, despite her earlier statement, she itemized other benefits. "I've become a much stronger person. I wouldn't be half as stubborn as I am. If I have a good day and do things, I don't take it for granted — to go out for coffee, or for wine or the cinema. I appreciate it so much more than someone who doesn't have an illness. I'm much more appreciative of a good day, and I really, really appreciate a good night's sleep."

Better Eating Habits

Patients mentioned that because of Crohn's disease or colitis, they became more conscious and careful about what they ate and how it affected their digestive systems. They were grateful to IBD for forcing them to do so.

Alisa has implemented a health transformation. "I don't know how else it would have come up," she said. "I would have never turned a spotlight on my health if it were not for colitis. I'd never cook. I wouldn't work out, and I'd drink a lot. For me, the upside is being a more well-rounded, healthy person. It's transformed how I approach life, how I eat. I'm grateful. If I could go back, I wouldn't want to have colitis, but the upside is improved health."

IBD has even kept some patients out of harm's way. Emmett, a professional jazz musician, would have hung out with people doing drugs and alcohol and probably would have joined them, but he can't afford to because he has Crohn's disease. His drugs are non-psychotropic. "I have to be very, very aware of my body and what I put into it," he said. "I'm a lot more cautious about what I eat. I don't drink or smoke or do any drugs, directly from having Crohn's. I would have done that if I didn't have it."

Dana said she has a better appreciation of health in general, and she credits her adherence to a rigid diet that has helped her ulcerative colitis. "This diet that I'm on is really strict and hard, and I would not choose to be on it," she said. "But the upside is, I can only put natural, whole foods into my body. I'll be the healthiest 90-year-old ever."

Creating Order

Colin enumerates the qualities he has acquired in order to take care of himself and his Crohn's. "It's made me more organized," he said. "I was not very good about setting a schedule, but I had to because of the disease. I had to make sure my medications were in order, that I got to my doctor's appointments, that I ate enough before I left the house, that I didn't just eat and run. I'm more adept at making a plan. I guess I can thank IBD in a way. It does make you grow up a little bit, makes you more mature, especially when I had it at 22 or 23, because you have to take charge of things other people my age don't have to take charge of: insurance, medical companies, doctors, medications. Instead of going out and drinking, partying, and having a good time, I was calling insurance companies."

Positive Rebellion

Some people described how they have accomplished more in their lives than they would have, just to prove that they are able do difficult things despite having IBD.

Adina started to talk slowly about the upside, as if she hadn't considered it before. "I'm much more in tune with my body than I would have been. I guess that's a positive," she said. And from there she was off and running. "I've been very overly driven, and that's possibly because, since I was diagnosed in college, I didn't want anyone to tell me I couldn't do anything. So I graduated in three years, did grad school in a year and a half, and I've been working since I was 20. This was probably all because of my illness."

Bob also reacted strongly when anyone told him he couldn't do something because of his Crohn's disease. "I was a high school wrestler because someone told me, 'You can't wrestle. You have Crohn's.' I stunk, but I wrestled. Once upon a time, I had a manager at a job when I was a sales assistant who told me I couldn't be a financial adviser. I studied psychology and sociology with a minor in criminal justice in school and became fascinated with finances. I went home and studied and became a financial adviser." Bob is now a vice president at a prestigious brokerage firm.

He wears an ostomy bag, has a family, and volunteers money and time on the Crohn's and Colitis Foundation.

Who says people with ostomies can't climb Mount Kilimanjaro or Mount Everest? Maybe nobody ever asked until Rob Hill, an ostomate, decided to lead treks up major mountains with others who have had an ostomy. Clinton, a 16-year-old Canadian who had been extremely ill with Crohn's, had a complete turnaround with the help of ostomy surgery and Humira. That was when he saw an invitation to climb Mount Kilimanjaro. The purpose of the trek was to dramatize the reality that people with ostomies can meet extreme mental and physical challenges. Coming out of a period when all he felt was weakness and helplessness, Clinton embraced the effort to scale the nearly 20,000-foot mountain. It took the party six days to reach the summit. He described how he did it.

"I'd never been in high altitudes before," he said. "I'd always wanted to speak out about the disease and bring awareness to it, and this seemed like the way. Rob whipped me into shape with a Marine Corps-type workout. I was mentally prepared and had to be physically prepared, and whatever happened after that was up to the mountain." The night they would climb the last section of the mountain was known as "summit night," Clinton said. "Rob warned us that this would be the hardest challenge," he said, reliving the experience as he spoke. That's when I started getting nervous. Now, it's go time. We got up at midnight to start climbing," he said. "You can't see what you are climbing, which is better in some sense since it's so steep and it's freezing. It's steep switchback trails straight up and a section of rock. I just kept looking at the feet [of other climbers] in front of me. The altitude was getting to me at that point. I puked once. That [climb] was the hardest physical challenge of my life. It took eight hours of nonstop hiking in the dark to reach the summit. We arrived at the perfect time — we saw the sun rising. It was absolutely beautiful. I had tears in my eyes. I couldn't believe I was there after going through so much."

Clinton said that he dealt well with the rudimentary washrooms in the area or the lack of them on the mountain. "The whole point was not to let IBD stop you," he said. "That was our tag line. When I reached the summit, it dawned on me that I was taking my life back. That was the big moment for me. I'll never forget it."

Carly, who had undergone surgery for an ostomy when she was only 10, followed Rob Hill up Mount Everest. She had met Hill at an event sponsored by the Intestinal Disease Education and Awareness Society of Canada. After the event, she said, Rob "messaged me one day and said, 'Carly, we're thinking of bringing you to Everest. Are you up for it?' I guess he just saw something in me," she said proudly. Carly, who was 17 when we spoke, has adjusted to her ostomy "and it's made me who I am," she said. "I feel kind of blessed to have it because of all the opportunities that have arisen from it."

During the trek, Carly climbed to the base camp, which was almost 17,600 feet up the 29,000–foot-high mountain, an accomplishment in itself, and she stayed there while some others climbed to the summit. Carly described the process of emptying an ostomy bag in the four-degrees-below-zero weather on Mount Everest. "We were all in tents, so you kind of want to do it really fast," she explained. "We had body wipes, so you'd sit or lie on them before you changed your ostomy [bag], so the wipes got warm. You'd put the ostomy [supplies] under your shirt so they were warm and you'd do it as fast as possible. We had garbage bags and everything is carried down by Sherpas [members of an ethnic group in eastern Nepal who help climbers on Everest.] The outhouse is made of rocks built over a big plastic barrel and they carry the barrel down, too.

"We did a side trek to a place called Kala Patther, which offers the best views of Everest," she continued. "But halfway up, I had to empty my ostomy bag, and I was kneeling, facing the rock. All the Sherpas were looking at me, wondering why I wasn't squatting." One of the Sherpas explained to the others what an ostomy bag is. "I came back and they asked if I could lift up my shirt to see it." She did. "One pointed and said, 'Haaahhh, and the other guy said, Aaaahhh.' It was so funny."

Dealing with Adversity

There's pride in knowing that you've dealt with something difficult and you are still standing. Having that awareness can enhance your self-esteem, even as you contemplate how hard it's been. "You've had to struggle for something," said Adam. "It can give you a sense of purpose." Adam added that he was not ready to consider any benefits of having Crohn's, saying, "It's dangerous to think of really negative things like chronic diseases as benevolent. Life would be better if I didn't have Crohn's. I don't think it's a blessing. But there is a sense of accomplishment and pride in dealing with something that's truly difficult. Though I've been very blessed in a lot of ways, sometimes you have to deal with very difficult things. You know your life hasn't been a cakewalk. It's nice to feel like you can confront adversity."

Morphing IBD into a Career

When I spoke with Maggie, the poster girl for ostomies mentioned in Chapter Twelve, she was happily studying in nursing school and thinking about her life. "I'd be a really boring person if I didn't have Crohn's," she said. "I don't know what I'd do with my life. I'd be one of those girls doing my makeup all the time. I feel better about myself because I have an ostomy. I'm thinking about being a stoma nurse, because I think people with the actual ostomy make better stoma nurses. I can't wait. I just want to help people with ostomies. Maybe it was meant to be part of my life, and I'm blessed to be embracing it."

Comparing Diseases

As has been mentioned earlier, one way to cope with IBD is to acknowledge that others are worse off and to feel grateful for the degree of disease you have. There is always someone who has it worse.

"I'd like to think I'm more mature because I've had to deal with Crohn's," said Charlotte, 15. "I think I handle certain crisis situations better. I can empathize with people more. Crohn's is bad, but there are things that are worse. There are kids that have cancer that may die. I'm not going to die of Crohn's. I'm kind of lucky."

Josh compared his IBD to his brother's severe autism. "His life is 100 times worse," he said. "He can't talk. He can't drive a car. He goes to school all year around. Crohn's made me stronger. I have an obstacle to overcome, but his obstacle is 10 times harder than mine. It's made me a stronger and a happier person."

Andrew suffered badly from Crohn's when he was diagnosed at age 21 and he underwent surgery for the removal of parts of his intestines, called a resection. Before that, he said, he "never gave a thought about what it would be like to have a major disability." That summer, not only couldn't he walk, he couldn't even lift his leg to get into the hospital bed. "It changed my outlook," he said. He added that he had never before felt helpless, nor had he needed to rely on others. "It's made me appreciate the illness, the hospital, the doctors. I can't believe it got that bad. I'm fortunate to get better. Some people don't. People have cancer when it's a terminal illness." Three years after his diagnosis, Andrew raised $5,000 and rode his bike from Baltimore to Portland, Oregon to support cancer research.

Crohn's also made a tougher person out of Tiffany. "I don't have a lot of medical freak-outs," she told me. "I don't worry about cancer or anything like that." In fact, after grappling with Crohn's, Tiffany professed to feel no fear about other life-threatening illnesses. "If I get something that kills me, I won't have died of Crohn's. Anything that kills me that's not Crohn's is a win for me. If Crohn's can't kill me, I've beaten Crohn's." In a sense, Tiffany has turned her illness into a kind of wrestling match that she will win no matter what.

Maturity

Many people interviewed said that, in one way or another, the experience of coping with IBD had given them a perspective beyond their years. That doesn't mean that people with IBD are smarter, wiser, or better people, but that in some corner of their lives, they know what it is to feel vulnerable and that, it is hoped, will translate into feeling compassion for other people at an age when many young people are largely self-absorbed. It means that people with IBD generally don't have the luxury of making stupid choices (even if they sometimes do.)

"Even when I was younger and sick in the hospital," said Benzion, "I remember relating to the whole situation as a challenge that ultimately offers something good. I didn't look at it as merely a pity situation, poor me, whatever. It was always a challenge that I had to step up to the plate to meet.

"I have a specific memory of going to a healer," he continued. "I must have been around 12, and he gave me homework that when I'm in pain, I should inhale the name of my God and then, on the exhale, say 'I love you.' Even at that age, doing it was powerful," he said. "That breathing exercise and that intention was very centering, grounding and calming. It caused me to be even more spiritual in general in my life. Socially, the people I was close to were getting into drugs, and I missed that whole scene, because I just wasn't around it. I matured a lot because of it. I got married at 19 and moved to a different country. I'm a much stronger person, more independent and mature. It wasn't like a near-death experience where I felt I needed to take charge of my life, but I've always been more of a serious person."

Susan, who was diagnosed with ulcerative colitis at 14, believes she was more mature in high school because of it. "I think I'm much more understanding of other people going through diseases," she said. "People open up to me, and I'm a pretty good listener. I make people comfortable, because you can't judge someone else when you're going to the bathroom 30 times a day in high school. It's made me a lot stronger. You have a hardship you're overcoming, and with that comes struggles and pride and success and perseverance."

Shawn admittedly has his whiny moments about having Crohn's disease. But he remembers something a friend told him when he was young: "Crohn's has made you the person you are today, and everybody loves you and thinks you have a wonderful personality." "That was wonderful to hear, of course," Shawn said years later. "My friends described me as an old soul even when I was younger. I was never the type to do idiotic or dangerous things. I do attribute having a milder personality to having Crohn's. I feel like I have this one life, and it might not go as far as others, and I'd better make the best of it. I just want to be happy. That's all I care about through all the pain. That's what I strive for. Having my friends and family happy around me makes me happy."

Elan has a considerable family history of IBD, so it would be natural if his father granted him a little latitude because of his Crohn's disease. Not so. In high school, Elan tutored bar- and bat-mitzvah students. One day, he was late for a lesson because he had to go to the bathroom. His dad chastised him, Elan said, saying, "'I do know how hard it is, but you have to factor in extra time to get places on time.' Other people would have given me a free pass on it," Elan said, "but the message I got was, 'I understand what you're going through, and you still need to be responsible for yourself, and this is who you are. You want to live with this rather than find an excuse to not do the things you want to do.' That was powerful and frustrating, because all you wanted was that excuse, but it wasn't available in my family."

General Outlook

For some, IBD has become so much a part of their identity that patients don't know who they would be without it. "I would be kind of upset if one day I didn't have Crohn's disease," said 18-year-old Sarah. "It would be weird, and I would have to make another adjustment again and find a different community." A Camp Oasis veteran, Sarah has many friends from the camp, and she has incorporated Crohn's into her identity "not in a negative way," she said. "It made me a lot better of a person. I used be really shy and awkward and not talk to adults. I was forced to do things out of my comfort zone and do things I didn't want to do. It made me a lot more straightforward and a lot more resilient. 'Resilient' is the favorite word for my mom and me. I felt I was more mature and had a different outlook than other people. It works out, really."

"I think Crohn's put me through a lot of hurting times, but I wouldn't change anything," said Krystal. "I was given a lot of opportunities because of it. I'd never have gone to camp and never have met the really important people in my life. I'd be a much different person if I didn't have all the medical things happen to me, and I didn't have all those chances. I think it made me into a better person."

Conclusion

Alisa articulated what many people with IBD may have felt, but couldn't express. She turned the negative aspects of having ulcerative colitis inside out and transformed them into positive qualities.

"A lot of us with ulcerative colitis [and Crohn's] are on fire, literally," she told me. "We're stubborn, fiery, independent, passionate, loving, beautiful creatures. Recognize that about yourself and take what you can from this disease. Find out who you are. Figure out the whole picture. Find the route out of this and really apply yourself to better yourself and heal yourself from the inside out."

Amen to that. If you are reading this and thinking that there is no way that you can do this, or that your disease is too overwhelming or too intractable, I'm here to tell you that you can identify something you *can* heal, whether it's a relationship or feelings inside that have gone yet unexpressed. By speaking your truth, you will have at least made it easier to come to terms with living your life as fully as possible with IBD. And that alone is a triumph.

REFERENCES

Akobeng, A., Miller, V., Firth, D., Suresh-Babu, M.V., Mir, P., Thomas, A. G., "Quality of Life of Parents and Siblings of Children with Inflammatory Bowel Disease," *Journal of Pediatric Gastroenterology and Nutrition* (1999), 28, S40-S42,

Amre, D.K., Lambrette, P., Law L., et al, "Investigating the Hygiene Hypothesis as a Risk Factor in Pediatric Onset Crohn's Disease: A Case-control Study," *The American Journal of Gastroenterology*, (2006) 101: 1005–1011. See www.ncbi.nim.nih.gov/pubmed/16573775.

Ananthakrishnan, Ashwin N., "Environmental Triggers for Inflammatory Bowel Disease," *Current Gastroenterology Reports* (January 2013), 15(1): 302. doi: 10.1007/s11894-012-0302-4, p.27. See www.ncbi.nim.gov/pmc/articles/PMC3537164/.

Cámara, Rafael J.A.; Gander, Marie-Louise; Begré, Stefan; Von Känel, Roland (Swiss Inflammatory Bowel Disease Cohort Study Group), "Post-traumatic Stress in Crohn's Disease and its Association with Disease Activity," *Frontline Gastroenterology* (2010),

Carpenter, Siri, "That Gut Feeling," American Psychological Association, *Monitor on Psychology* (September 2012), Vol. 43, No. 8. See www.apa.org/monitor/2012/09/gut-feeling.aspx.

Crohn, B.B., Ginzburg L., Oppenheimer, G.D., "Regional Ileitis: A Pathological and Clinical Entity," *JAMA* (1932), 99: 1323–1329.

Eagleman, Dr. David, "'Incognito': What's Hiding in the Unconscious Mind." See www.npr.org/2011/05/31/136495499/incognito-whats-hiding-in-the-unconscious-mind.

Ekbom, Anders, "The Epidemiology of IBD: A Lot of Data but Little Knowledge. How shall we proceed?" See onlinelibrary.wiley.com, John Wiley & Sons, Dec. 14, 2006, and *Inflammatory Bowel Diseases* Vol. 10, No., 7, pp. S32–S34, February 2004.

Engstrom, Dr. Ingemar, "Psychological Problems in Siblings of Children and Adolescents with Inflammatory Bowel Disease," *European Child and Adolescent Psychiatry*, Vol. 1, No. 1, January 1992.

Frei, Rosemary, "Alternative Medicine Use Common in Pediatric IBD," *Gastroenterology and Endoscopy News*, February 2009. Jolley, Christopher: Commentary www.gastroendonews.com/ViewArticle.aspx?d_id=190&a_id=12571.

Gray, Wendy N., "Parenting Stress in Pediatric IBD: Relations with Child Psychopathology, Family Functioning, and Disease Severity," (May 1, 2014), Journal of Developmental and Behavioral Pediatrics. 2013 May; 34(4): 237–244.

Hommel, Kevin A.; Denson, Lee A.; Crandall, Wallace V.; Mackner, Laura M., "Behavioral Functioning and Treatment Adherence in Pediatric Inflammatory Bowel Disease," *Journal of Gastroenterology and Hepatology*, (November 2008), 4(11): 785–791.

Hordvik, Ellen, "Sick Children in the Family." See www.bufetat.no/Documents/Bufetat.no/Program%20for%20foreldrerettleiing/Temahefte/Sick%20children%20in%20the%20family.pdf.

Kane, Sunanda. "What Physicians Don't Know about Patient Dietary Beliefs and Behavior Can Make a Difference," *Expert Review of Gastroenterology & Hepatology,* September 2012, Vol. 6, No. 5 , Pages 545-547
Read More: http://informahealth-care.com/doi/abs/10.1586/egh.12.43

Langholz, Ebbe, "Current Trends in Inflammatory Bowel Disease: The Natural History," *Therapeutic Advances in Gastroenterology* (March 2010), 3(2): 77–86.

Levitan, Hayley, "Advocation for Children with Crohn's Disease and Ulcerative Colitis" (2011). See www.education.com/reference/article/advocation-for-children-crohns-colitis/.

Lal, Simon; Prasad, Neeraj; Ryan, Manijeh; Tangri, Sabrena; Silverberg, M.S.; Gordon, A.; Steinhart, H., "Cannabis Use Amongst Patients with Inflammatory Bowel Disease," *European Journal of Gastroenterology & Hepatology* (2011).

Lindberg, Annellie; Ebbeskog, Brit; Karlen, Per; Oxelmark, Lena, "Inflammatory Bowel Disease Professionals' Attitudes to and Experiences of Complementary and Alternative Medicine," *BMC Complementary & Alternative Medicine* (2013), 13:349. See www.biomedcentral.com/1472-6882/13/349.

Mackner, Laura M.; Crandall Wallace V.; Szigethy, Eva M., "Psychosocial Functioning in Pediatric Inflammatory Bowel Disease," *The Journal of Pediatric Psychology,* 2006 Mar;12(3):239-44.

McHale, Susan M.; Updegraff Kimberly A.; Whiteman, Shawn D., "Sibling Relationships and Influences in Childhood and Adolescence," *Journal of Marriage and Family 74,* (October 2012), 913 – 930.

"Transitioning a Patient With IBD From Pediatric to

Adult Care," on the website of NASPGHAN, the North American Society for Pediatric Gastroenterology, Hepatology and Nutrition. See http://www.naspghan.org/files/documents/pdfs/medical-resources/ibd/Checklist_PatientandHealthcarePro diver_TransitionfromPedtoAdult.pdf.

Oliva-Hemker, Maria; Ziring, David; Bousvaros, Athos, editors, "Your Child with Inflammatory Bowel Disease: A Family Guide for Caregiving" (Hepatology and Nutrition North American Society for Pediatric Gastroenterology, 2010).

Lindfred, Helene; Saalman, Robert; Nillsson, S.; Reichenberg, Kjell, "Inflammatory Bowel Disease and Self-esteem in Adolescence," *Acta Pædiatrica* (2007).

Reigada, Laura C.; McGovern, Amanda; Tudor, Megan E;, Walder, Deborah J., "Collaborating with Pediatric Gastroenterologists to Treat Co-Occurring Inflammatory Bowel Disease and Anxiety in Pediatric Medical Settings," *Cognitive and Behavioral Practice*, Volume 21, Issue 4, November 2014, Pages 372–385.

Reigada, L. C., Benkov, K. J., Bruzzese, J.M., Hoogendoorn, C., Szigethy, E., Briggie, A., Walder, D.J., Warner, Masia C., "Integrating Illness, Concerns into Cognitive Behavioral Therapy for Children and Adolescents with Inflammatory Bowel Disease and Co-occurring Anxiety," *Journal for Nurses in Specialty Practice*, (2013), 18(2), 133-143.

Reigada, L. C., Bruzzese, J.M., Benkov, K. J. Levy, J., Waxman, A.R., Petkova, E., Warner, Masia, C., "Illness-specific Anxiety: Implications for IBD-related Functioning and Medical Usage in Youth with Inflammatory Bowel Disease," *Journal for Nurses in Specialty Practice*, (2011). 16(3), 207-215.

Rubin, Hannah, "Crohn's Is on the Rise Among Children," *Jewish Daily Forward*, August 14, 2012. See forward.com/articles/160724/crohns-is-on-the-rise-among-children/?p=all.

Szigethy, Eva, McLafferty, Laura, Goyal, Alka, "Inflammatory Bowel Disease," *Child & Adolescent Psychiatric Clinics of North America* (2011), 58, 903-920

Tresca, Amber J., "Who Gets IBD? Certain Ages and Ethnicities Have a Higher Risk of Developing IBD" (2015). ibdcrohns.about.com/od/diagnostictesting/p/ibdepidemology.htm.

Acknowledgements

Years ago, I confided in a friend who had published her own book of nonfiction with a major publishing house, that I'd always wanted to write a book. I wanted to leave a legacy, I told her. "Make a quilt, it's a lot easier," was her reply.

Now that I have run — or, rather, slowly walked — through my own gauntlet of writing a book about a subject I've been living with and thinking about for years, I have many people to thank. Cindy Barrilleaux, my editor, was good-natured and extremely efficient. She set the pace for my writing and made excellent suggestions. I am forever grateful for her help.

I am also grateful to Emily Zammitti, a student at the Drexel University School of Public Health, who analyzed my data, searched for academic articles and did it all with commitment and good cheer. I am filled with gratitude for my husband, Jake, who carefully read the manuscript and offered wise advice. I am grateful for my writing group: Rabbi Dayle Friedman, Sonia Voynow, Meredith Barber and Sandy Kosmin, who helped guide me throughout the process of writing this book. My good friend Deborah McKnight also offered excellent guidance and provided a patient ear. My sons, Daniel and Ezra, could always distract me when I needed a break.

.